45 Ways to Live Like an Italian

ITALIAN-INSPIRED SELF-CARE TRADITIONS for EVERYDAY HAPPINESS

RAELEEN D'AGOSTINO MAUTNER, PhD

sourcebooks

To Aldo Signorello and Dino Signorello,
my fellow musicians of ENTERPRISE.

Copyright © 2023 by Raeleen D'Agostino Mautner
Cover and internal design © 2023 by Sourcebooks
Cover design © Kimberly Glyder
Cover and internal illustration © Kimberly Glyder
Internal design by Lindsey Cleworth

This publication is designed to provide accurate and authoritative information in regard to the subject matter covered. It is sold with the understanding that the publisher is not engaged in rendering legal, accounting, or other professional service. If legal advice or other expert assistance is required, the services of a competent professional person should be sought. —*From a Declaration of Principles Jointly Adopted by a Committee of the American Bar Association and a Committee of Publishers and Associations*

This book is not intended as a substitute for medical advice from a qualified physician. The intent of this book is to provide accurate general information in regard to the subject matter covered. If medical advice or other expert help is needed, the services of an appropriate medical professional should be sought.

All brand names and product names used in this book are trademarks, registered trademarks, or trade names of their respective holders. Sourcebooks is not associated with any product or vendor in this book.

Published by Sourcebooks
P.O. Box 4410, Naperville, Illinois 60567-4410
(630) 961-3900
sourcebooks.com

Cataloging-in-Publication Data is on file with the Library of Congress.

Printed and bound in China.
OGP 10 9 8 7 6 5 4 3 2 1

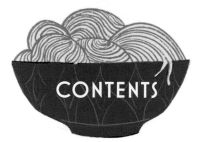

CONTENTS

The Italian Celebration of Self

The Italian Celebration of Relationships

The Italian Celebration of Beliefs

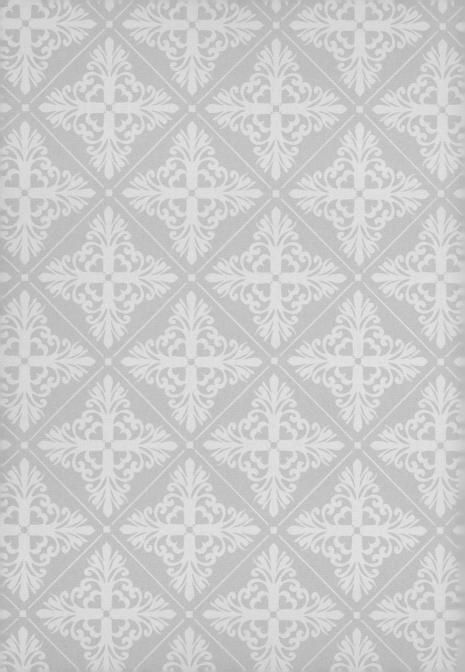

INTRODUCTION

The Italian Celebration of La Dolce Vita

Author Luigi Barzini once described Italy as having the capacity to be "gay, tragic, mad, pastoral, archaic, modern, or **simply *dolce*.**" Thus, when you imagine Italy, you might think of Renaissance genius, the Roman army's invincibility, revered saints, dedicated artisans, insightful philosophers, or brilliant inventors who gave the world everything from musical notation to the microscope and too much more to mention. And, of course, you would be right. Italy is all that. Italy is also synonymous with exquisite food, unparalleled wines, thermal springs, sunlit fields, innovative cinematography, confident women, and suave, well-dressed men. We can't argue with that either.

However, there is one Italian cultural element that doesn't receive nearly as much press as the aforementioned, because rather than being a tangible representation, it is a philosophical mindset of the Italian approach to life. It is the "simply dolce" description in Barzini's phrase, which we will examine more closely in this book. Regardless of the political and bureaucratic reasons for which Italians may admit they are disgruntled in the land that Petrarch named "the *bel paese*" back in the fourteenth century, on a daily, more personal level, the concept of "la dolce vita," or the sweet life, refers to the ability to savor simple pleasures throughout the course of an ordinary day. In Parma (home of the renowned Parmigiano Reggiano cheese, prosciutto di Parma, and the Duchess Maria Luigia's Violetta di Parma fragrance), a commonly used expression in local dialect captures this lifestyle philosophy beautifully: *Tola su dölsa*. Roughly translated, it means to take things sweetly and stay calm.

For Italians, the sweet life, or la dolce vita, is the experience of sipping a morning cappuccino while looking out over the balcony toward a brilliant sunrise. It is the aroma of long-simmering tomato sauce that welcomes you into the kitchen like a warm hug. It is the distant gong of the *campana della chiesa*, the church bell, reminding you that the gift of life at all stages has value and meaning. Living a dolce vita (in contrast to the aimlessly over-indulgent plight of Marcello Mastroianni's character in the famous 1960 Fellini film) doesn't require wealth, status, luxury possessions, or even a villa on the Mediterranean. It just requires immersing yourself in the small details of your day, refusing to speed through your experiences at someone else's frenetic pace, and finding purpose in every task worthy of your attention. A dolce vita lifestyle beckons you to slow your pace and enjoy the happy moments wherever you find them.

Living the Italian dolce vita is not about pretending that hardships don't exist. Despite a healthy distrust of politics, skepticism toward the church, frustration over high taxes, few jobs in a hurting economy, and the ongoing corruption of organized crime in the south, at the heart of every Italian is the *arte di arrangiarsi* (literally the art of getting by) when faced with situations that threaten well-being. *Arrangiarsi* means that amid challenges will come an even stronger determination to make the best of reality. One can find respite in the warmth of family, friends, laughter, good food, local wine, or evening *passeggiate* (strolls) along the town square.

Life for all of us can be pretty stressful at times. We might turn on the TV news only to be bombarded with horrific images of war, predictions of economic disaster, reports of upticks in violent crime, or a killer pandemic that has probably already affected your life or the life of someone you care about. You might call a friend to say "Hello" and instead of enjoying pleasant chitchat, you get sucked into a political argument that results in a rift between the two of you because you don't agree. Perhaps you get a call from your doctor asking you to schedule a follow-up test because something didn't look right on your previous X-ray. The Italian *arte di arrangiarsi* is there for you too. It is the confidence to know you will get by and the ability to redirect your energy toward the many positive aspects of your life.

✒

Roman philosopher Marcus Aurelius believed that we have the power to control our own happiness to the extent that we can control our thoughts. While there may be some external situations that cannot be changed, there are some ways we *can* have an impact. We can make improvements to our health, attitude, mood, appearance, physical surroundings, and relationships.

I have observed the dolce vita firsthand throughout the years—from my own extended Italian family, from my relatives who reside in Italy, from my experiences studying and conducting cross-cultural research in Italy throughout the years, and through my presentations with Italian audiences, who talked openly to me about aspects of their daily lives that bring them pleasure. The dolce vita is a lifestyle philosophy that has helped hundreds of readers of my earlier book, *Living La Dolce Vita*, make life richer, more enjoyable, and less stressful. Italian lifestyle traditions are about self-care. They teach us that sometimes we have to give ourselves a break from negativity, let go of small arguments, and stay focused on thinking and doing that which brings us happiness and enhances our well-being.

If you have ever been to Italy, the transformative nature of the *bel paese* has certainly wound its way into your soul. But you don't have to visit Italy to live like an Italian or to celebrate life like an Italian. The ideas I lay out in this book can help you reduce stress and enjoy more of your life regardless of your age, economic status, ethnicity, race, religion, gender, or geography. A *fai da te* (do-it-yourself) section follows each chapter and offers ways to apply the ideas throughout the book. *45 Ways to Live Like an Italian* will inspire you to adopt the sweetness of Italy and begin to notice the small daily details that turn what you might once have considered ordinary moments into extraordinary experiences that are worthy of celebration.

To that end, I wish you ***buon leggere* (happy reading)!**

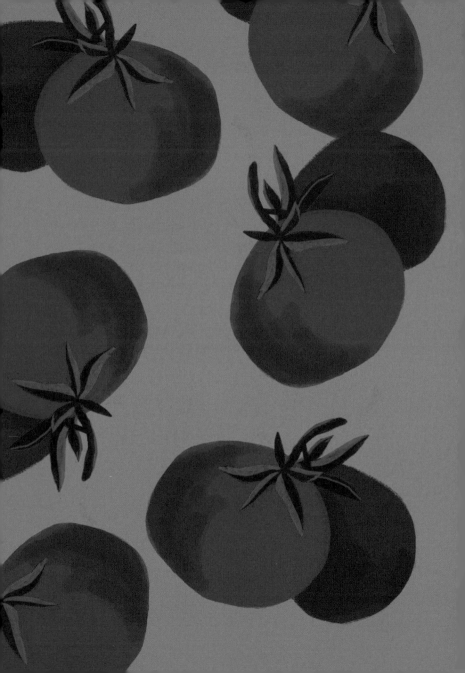

The Italian Celebration of Food

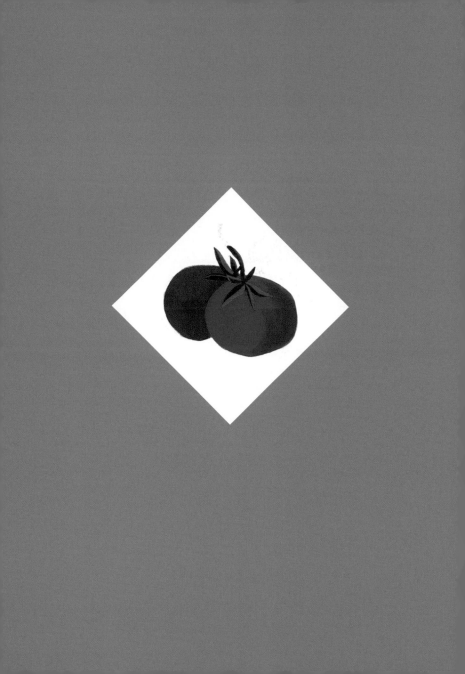

1

Mangia Bene

Eating Well, the Italian Way

Mangia! It is one of the most important Italian commands, whether verbalized by parents to children, adults to their friends, or family members to each other. Italians are serious about their food. They don't fool around when it comes to what, how, and with whom they eat. The emphasis on eating well goes at least as far back as Renaissance times, when Leonardo da Vinci wrote in his *Notebooks*: "In order to stay in optimal health, eat only when you want and relish food; chew thoroughly that it may do you good; have it well-cooked, unspiced and undisguised; and let your food—rather than medicine—be your source of wellness." We have all heard of how influential sound nutrition is on physical wellness, but increasingly we are learning how important an impact it has on mental health, especially in alleviating symptoms of anxiety and depression.

The Mediterranean diet, as we now call it, was originally associated with Ancel Keys, a physiologist at the University of Minnesota. In 1951, Keys was giving a lecture at the first Congress of the Food and Agriculture Organization of the United Nations after World War II when one attendee, a doctor named Gino Bergami from the University Hospital of Naples, commented on Keys's observation of the high incidences of cardiac death in the United States among men ages thirty to fifty-nine. Bergami told Keys that cardiovascular disease was extremely uncommon in his hospital and later invited Keys to come check for himself.

Keys's biologist wife, Margaret Haney, immediately began collecting and analyzing blood samples of Neapolitan steelworkers, comparing them with the samples of men in Minnesota. They discovered a significant difference in cholesterol levels, which could partially explain the difference in heart attack rates. But Keys and Haney became fascinated with an even broader, more holistic definition of the Mediterranean diet, which went beyond an eating style based on fresh fruits and vegetables, whole grains, legumes, and nuts, with moderate to sparing use of olive oil, dairy, and wine and limited inclusion of meats and sweets. Also important was a practice of eating together with family and friends, walking or bicycling daily, and coming together in community venues like parish churches for group prayer.

While research on Mediterranean dietary patterns has consistently demonstrated its preventative effect on cardiovascular disease, type 2 diabetes, high blood pressure, inflammation, high cholesterol, and other diseases, equally important is its effect on mental health and overall well-being. A Mediterranean nutritional approach may actually influence our affect or emotional landscape—how we view the world in which we live. For example, when archival data of the dietary habits of over nine thousand Adventist Church attendees were examined, researchers found that those who ate more Mediterranean-type foods had more positive and less negative emotions than did those who ate a typical Western diet.

The Mediterranean diet has also been shown to be helpful in cases of depression and anxiety. In a recent literature review on the benefits of the Mediterranean diet, results of several studies showed a greater reversal of depressive symptoms, even when compared to a social support control group, in those who adhered to a Mediterranean diet. In yet another study, the Mediterranean diet was shown to have a protective effect from the typical stressors of student academic life. In a cross-sectional sample of 502 students at the University of Turin, those who reported greater adherence to a Mediterranean diet had more positive attitudes and overall better mental health.

Finally, even young people seem to feel happier when eating Mediterranean-style cuisine. In a population of 527 adolescents in Spain, more subjective happiness and higher quality of life scores were reported in those with a greater adherence to the Mediterranean diet.

It is hardly surprising that in 2010, UNESCO recognized the Mediterranean diet as an Intangible Heritage of Humanity, and in 2012, it was included as one of the most sustainable diets on the planet by the Food and Agriculture Organization. Besides having numerous physical and mental health benefits, it may also promote longevity. Ancel Keys lived to be one hundred, and his wife reached the age of ninety-seven.

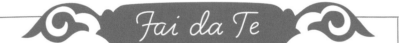

Fai da Te

GIVE THE MEDITERRANEAN DIET A TRY

The Mediterranean diet is about simple, life-affirming, fresh, seasonal foods. When you feed your body better, you not only feel better physically but, as we've just seen, you might also start to feel happier. If you want to give this healthy and delicious way of eating a try, here are a few ways to get started:

❄ Search for and download a free copy of the Mediterranean diet pyramid on the internet.

❄ Purchase a basic Italian cookbook that keeps to authentic Italian cuisine.

- ❄ Stock your pantry and fridge with the Italian fundamentals: whole-grain pasta, San Marzano tomatoes, extra virgin olive oil (the best you can afford), balsamic vinegar, oregano, garlic, and fresh basil.

- ❄ Keep lots of colorful produce on hand: eggplant, tomatoes, arugula, broccoli rabe, fresh basil, flat parsley. Also, if you eat dairy, choose fresh mozzarella and imported Parmigiano Reggiano.

- ❄ Shop seasonal produce at local markets whenever possible. In the past few years, Italians have given emphasis to the term "zero kilometer," which conveys their preference for food that has not traveled far from its source. There is also a nostalgic desire for local ingredients and dishes when family members move away from their hometown. It is not uncommon to load up with locally sourced foods and wines when they come back home for visits.

- ❄ Try making *homemade Italian tomato sauce* (recipe below), and invite family, friends, or neighbors to enjoy it with you. *This* recipe is an adaptation of an old recipe I found with a few added twists based on watching my grandmother at the stove. If you are a meat eater, of course, you can brown the meat or meatballs in a bit of olive oil in the same dutch oven you will then make the sauce in, and let the meat finish cooking in the simmering tomato liquid.

Homemade Italian Tomato Sauce

INGREDIENTS

2 (28-oz) cans whole tomatoes with basil, preferably San Marzano
(you can also use two containers of Pomì Italian crushed
tomatoes with basil)

A couple drizzles extra virgin olive oil (or water or low-sodium
vegetable broth)

1 yellow onion, minced

2 to 4 cloves garlic, peeled and minced

Splash of red wine or balsamic vinegar (optional)

Salt and pepper to taste

Pinch of dried oregano or Italian seasoning

A few fresh basil leaves, torn

DIRECTIONS

Place the tomatoes in a large bowl, and crush using your hands or
a potato masher. Remove and discard any hard cores from stem
ends and any skin and tough membranes. Set aside.

Place the oil (or water or low-sodium broth if you prefer) in a
large saucepan over medium-low heat. Add the onion, and cook
until soft and just beginning to brown, stirring with a wooden
spoon, about 3 minutes. Stir in the garlic, and cook until just
golden but not brown. Stir in the tomatoes and wine or vinegar.
Season with salt and pepper. Add the oregano. Bring to a boil;
then immediately reduce heat to low, and simmer until slightly
thickened, for about 2 to 3 hours, stirring occasionally.

When the sauce is almost done, stir in the basil; then continue cooking for 2 to 3 minutes more. Remove from heat and serve over hot pasta of your choice. If you have added meat to cook in the sauce, remove it to a separate plate. Then serve the pasta first as a *primo piatto* (first course), then the meat as a *secondo piatto* (second course), then finally an *insalata verde* (green salad) to cleanse the palate.

NOTE: If you are making the pasta at the same time as you make the sauce, you may add a ladle or two of the salted pasta water (when pasta is almost ready to be drained) to the tomato sauce if you prefer a thinner consistency.

La Dieta Flexitariana

Variations on Mediterranean Eating

From 2014 to 2022, the number of Italians who opted for a vegan lifestyle approximately doubled. While the health benefits of the Mediterranean diet are undisputed, mounting evidence now suggests that a vegan, whole-food, low-fat, plant-based approach to eating may improve overall health. Some research is also finding that eating a whole-food, plant-based diet improves both mood and productivity through a decrease in anxiety, depression, and stress and an improvement in focus.

Remember that eating more nutritionally dense foods is a gesture of holistic self-care aimed at nurturing your body, mind, and spirit. Of course, whatever choice you make regarding eating style should be solely between you and your physician, but it always pays to do your research and read the studies as well. Remember there are also junk-food vegans and vegetarians who essentially do no better in preserving their health than if they just continued to eat animals, dairy, and extracted oils. They may eliminate the burgers but still eat chips and candy bars and drink sodas and other substances that the body doesn't even recognize as nutrition.

A whole-food, plant-based, salt-, oil-, and sugar-free lifestyle diet has helped many people optimize their health and have more energy. Some choose this path out of concern for the environment (we know that meat consumption is responsible for releasing greenhouse gases such as methane, carbon dioxide, and nitrous oxide, which experts say contribute to climate change). Others choose to go vegan for ethical or empathetic reasons.

Interestingly, even more Americans (6 percent) are gravitating toward a vegan lifestyle than are Italians (2 percent), but one thing is certain: as more research is published about the benefits, the plant-based lifestyle is slowly gaining momentum everywhere. One of the lesser-known facts pertaining to dietary habits is that nutrients influence mental states.

A vegan Mediterranean diet still emphasizes the importance of physical activity throughout the day and drinking plenty of water. It also allows generous amounts of whole-food or whole-grain starches, such as whole wheat pasta, potatoes, rice, polenta, legumes, beans, fruits, and vegetables. Seeds, nuts, avocados, and whole olives, although healthy, are only to be eaten sparingly because of their high fat content. Desserts are only an occasional treat, not a daily habit; preferably they are sweetened not with refined sugar but with whole dates, ripe bananas, maple syrup, or unsweetened applesauce.

Some Italians practice a hybrid of traditional Mediterranean and vegan Mediterranean eating styles. A recent article in the online publication *Il Giornale del Cibo* referred to a growing number of Italians identifying themselves as following a *dieta flexitariana*, or a flexible diet, that was neither strictly vegan nor entirely vegetarian. This way of eating emphasized primarily fresh produce but did not entirely eliminate the occasional egg, meat, fish, and dairy.

Whatever degree of the Mediterranean diet you decide to adopt, you will surely get far more benefits than you would if you continue to (over)eat the standard American diet.

HOW TO EXPLORE HEALTHY VARIATIONS
ON THE CLASSIC MEDITERRANEAN DIET

Italy, like the rest of the world, is seeing a growing number of its people adopt a vegan lifestyle, one that excludes all animal products. Yet Italians are not about to completely abandon their familial Mediterranean cuisine. Here are some ways to explore a vegan approach to the traditional Italian diet.

❀ Search for a cookbook or YouTube channel that helps you explore vegan or vegetarian Italian recipes. I wasn't surprised to find there are not that many resources available for learning about these modifications on a Mediterranean diet, but I did find one cookbook that I use myself, written by Dominic Marro and Terri Marro Rinchik: *Plant-Based Italiano: Tradition Can Survive a Whole Food Plant-Based Diet*. What makes this collection special is that the recipes are not only based on whole-food vegan ingredients but they are also oil-free. In the introduction, Dominic explains how much maintaining his Italian heritage meant to him while at the same time wanting to find ways to make the traditional Italian dishes even healthier.

❀ Modify your favorite family recipes to make them meatless, completely vegan, or vegan and oil-free. Many Italian dishes of the *cucina povera* are already meatless, such as *pasta e fagioli*, *pasta e ceci*, *pasta e patate*, *fagioli e patate*, and Italian frittata (if you choose to eat eggs).

  – Make homemade tomato marinara sauce instead of Bolognese meat sauce. Pour over whole-grain pasta, and make a side salad filled with several types of greens (Italians love arugula, endive, red cabbage, black kale—*cavolo nero*—etc.), tomato, shredded carrots, celery, green onions (chives), mushrooms sautéed in a good balsamic vinegar, and a few imported Italian olives.

- For a low-fat salad dressing, start with a handful of walnuts, the juice of one lemon, one clove of fresh garlic, black pepper, and a pinch of salt (optional), and add water to thin it out to the consistency of a nice creamy dressing.

- As an appetizer, you can have a delicious bruschetta by slicing some crusty bread (optional: you can spray it lightly on both sides with an olive oil spray) and toasting it in the oven for a few minutes, making sure to turn it over to toast both sides. Top with some mashed avocado that has been combined with garlic powder, onion powder, oregano, and black pepper. For a lower-fat version, top with chopped ripe grape tomatoes that have been tossed with minced garlic, onion powder, black pepper to taste, oregano, and chopped fresh basil leaves. The possibilities are endless.

3

La Pasta Funzionale

Pasta with a Function

According to survey data, 98 percent of Italians love pasta, and six out of ten Italians eat this comfort food every day; this was especially true during the COVID-19 lockdown in 2020. Unfortunately, pasta has gotten a bad rap, nutritionally speaking, in the wake of the high-protein/low-carb craze. But pasta and other carbohydrates can provide an important source of energy for humans, and as it turns out, pasta can also make us feel happier! In one study, the roles of protein, fat, and carbohydrates were examined with respect to mood. Participants' food intake, including energy and nutrient composition, was calculated mathematically, and they also rated their mood after each meal over the course of nine days. While high protein consumption was correlated with greater depression, the opposite was true of carbohydrate intake.

Despite a gradual decline in pasta consumption with the rise of diverse ethnic food availability, Italians are still the largest consumers of pasta, and the benefits of a nice *spaghettata di mezzanotte* (midnight spaghetti snack) go far beyond lifting our spirits. Italians also continue to have significantly lower levels of obesity than in other parts of the Western world, and the statistics haven't changed much since I conducted my own cross-cultural research on the United States, England, and Italy.

Research has also found that higher pasta intake may be significantly associated with reduced long-term risk of stroke and atherosclerotic cardiovascular disease. As compared to other forms of carbohydrates from different sources, whole-grain pasta was found to have a lower glycemic index as well as glycemic load.

All this would lead us to think that pasta is the perfect food just as is—right? What could be more wholesome than the simple two-ingredient combination of semolina flour and water, shaped, dried, and eager to welcome a delicate plum tomato sauce, a healthful decoration of *aglio e olio* (garlic and oil), or dropped into a steaming broth with beans and veggies on a cold winter's day?

Enter the concept of "functional," or fortified pasta, promising the ability to lower cholesterol, stave off diabetes, and help us live even healthier lives. In turn, because of the bidirectionality of physical health and mental health, feeling better physically goes hand in hand with feeling emotionally more positive. Could the value of traditional pasta really be improved by adding nonconventional ingredients to the dough? Maybe, if we consider that "functional" pasta aims not only to improve the nutritional value of our favorite comfort food but also brings us an uplifting feeling, knowing that our functional pasta purchase helps defend the environment by using parts of foods that would normally be discarded. Additionally, it may also have the benefit of offering more choices that attract family and friends back to the dinner table.

Some additions to functional pasta dough consist of "upcycled" ingredients that would normally go to waste, such as the pulp from juicing, the oats extracted from oat milk, fish byproducts, etc. Other manufacturers are making functional pasta with *Opuntia ficus-indica* (prickly pear), which Italy is the second highest producer of globally. This cactus is said to contain a number of vitamins and minerals and may be beneficial in helping prevent hypercholesterolemia, diabetes, obesity, arteriosclerosis, and cardiovascular disease. You may also notice the popularity of "high protein" pasta made with a mixture of wheat, lentils, or pea protein.

Survey data indicates that those with higher levels of education and income are the most likely consumers of novel pasta products. Traditionalists are less likely to purchase functional pasta and often insist that the wheat their pasta is made from should be grown in their native Italy. (The reality is that much of the wheat in the better-known, mass-produced brands is imported.)

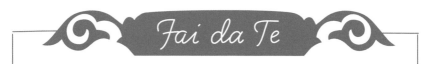

Fai da Te

HOW TO MAKE PASTA FUNCTION FOR YOU

No matter which side of the pasta/functional pasta divide you fall on, there are ways to explore some of the new pasta products you find at the supermarket, possibly increase the nutritional value of traditional pasta, and offer the kind of variety that sparks interest and brings more friends and family to the table. Here are some tips:

- ❀ Once a month, try a new type of pasta, and invite one or two relatives or friends you haven't seen in a while to the culinary adventure.

- ❀ Pay attention to portion sizes. Italians eat much smaller portions than we do in the United States. If you take time to savor each bite, you will hardly notice you are eating less.

- ❀ Make your own tomato sauce. Most jarred sauces contain way too much oil, sugar, and salt. You have total control over what you put in when you go back to the days when the aroma of simmering sauce fragranced the entire kitchen.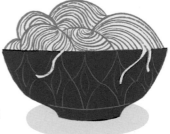

- ❀ Replace some of the pasta on your plate with vegetables and beans.

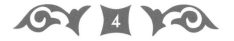

L'Alimentazione Sarda

Eat Like a Sardinian for a Long Life

Author Dan Buettner's research on "blue zones" explored the common habits he discovered among the five or so geographical areas throughout the world where an unusually high number of people live vibrant lives up to age one hundred or older. The behaviors of the centenarians included staying active (principally through walking), socializing, practicing one's faith, and eating mostly a plant-based Mediterranean diet, or rather a Sardinian diet, which seems to have health protective elements for both women *and* men. Whereas most centenarians around the world are disproportionately women (four to one), researchers discovered something unexpected in a little village called Villagrande Strisaili in Sardinia. In addition to its comparatively higher percentage of centenarians, there were an equal number of women and men living extraordinarily long lives. In their article published in the *Journal of Aging Research*, researchers Michel Poulain, Gianni Pes, and Luisa Salaris found that multiple factors were responsible for this Sardinian phenomenon. One of the factors that had a strong influence on emotional well-being and life satisfaction well into old age was positive social relationships.

Perceived health was another factor that influenced well-being in older Sardinians. Besides staying active much of the day, what they chose to eat played an important role in staying healthy. The red wine Sardinians drink from the mountaintop regions in Sardinia, for instance, had higher levels of polyphenols than most other wine. Made from grenache grapes, Sardinian Cannonau wine can actually be found in your local imported wine shop for very little money. Also, the milk of the cheeses Sardinians eat comes from grass-fed, not corn-fed, animals. Much of the food in the Sardinian "blue zone" is locally grown, and neither men nor women in Sardinia experience obesity as compared to those in the rest of Europe.

The Sardinian diet is not only about what it contains but what it does not (pesticides, hormones, dyes, sugars). As with the more general Mediterranean diet, the typical Sardinian menu consists of lots of vegetables, salads, vegetable-bean soups, and greens. In addition, they consume goat's and sheep's milk products (the cheeses made from these milks have been found to lower bad cholesterol as well as have anti-inflammatory properties), and they are also particular about their bread. Sardinian flatbread, or *carta di musica*, is made of high-protein, low-gluten triticum whole grain, which is the main ingredient in Italian pasta. Sardinian sourdough bread (*moddizzosu*) contains the healthy kind of bacteria and is easier to digest. Finally, their barley bread (made from barley flour, which you can make yourself in a high-powered mixer) is low on the glycemic index, and barley is also widely used to mop up the final drops of the typical Sardinian vegetable soups. These soups will most often contain fennel (the celery-like vegetable with an anise flavor) as well as fava beans, chickpeas, and tomatoes. Meat, just as in the more general Mediterranean diet, is used sparingly, and milk thistle tea, thought to clean the liver, is enjoyed on a daily basis.

Fai da Te

FOUR LIFESTYLE TIPS FOR SARDINIAN LONGEVITY

While geographical location plays a part in what makes Sardinia a "blue zone," it is only one factor. You don't need to live there to walk more, eat more healthily, and socialize more. It is never too late to build these positive lifestyle habits into each day. Here are some ways to do that:

Strengthen your relationships. Loneliness and isolation have come to the forefront as a result of a pandemic that no one initially knew how to cope with. Many workers began to work from home in 2020 and have stayed remote. Large gatherings were discouraged, and friends began losing contact with each other. Now is the time, while still staying safe, to begin reestablishing ties with family and friends. Find ways to reach out and make plans to go for a walk or enjoy a meal together. Expand your social network by joining a community garden, going back to your place of worship, or reviving the old Italian tradition of family (or friends) for Sunday dinner.

Grow some of your own food. Sardinians love to garden and grow their own fresh vegetables. They also like to forage for wild asparagus, wild greens (for salads), berries, and mushrooms (don't do this yourself without the proper training). They can and store surplus produce in their cellars. If you don't already have a garden, try allotting a small plot of land for growing the Italian basics: lettuce, tomatoes, basil, parsley, and squash. You can also grow these few items in pots if you don't have a garden space. There is nothing like the vibrant flavors of food that is eaten shortly after being harvested.

Learn to love cooking at home. Sardinians love to cook. Get used to the fact that if you want to optimize good health, you need to fall back in love with your kitchen stove. Take the time to enjoy the sounds of chopping onions, mincing garlic, and crushing fresh tomatoes for a delicious Sunday sauce. What you put into your body matters for your physical and mental well-being. You can gradually ease into the habit of cooking at home. If you work full-time, take advantage of weekends to do some batch cooking or meal prep to last two or three days during the week. Instead of looking at cooking as a chore, relax and enjoy the process. Invite the family to help with the cleanup or preparation, or invite a friend over to share the fun over a glass of Sardinian wine (Cannonau).

Move more. Sardinians stay active all day long. Physical activity, whether scheduling segments of exercise or simply moving around during the day, has been strongly correlated to greater levels of happiness. Staying active does not require a gym membership, nor cluttering one's home with big, heavy exercise machines. The Sardinian people in this area herd their sheep, milk their goats, forage for wild greens, cook, clean, and garden. They are in constant movement throughout the day. While you will most likely not be herding sheep or foraging for mushrooms, you can still find ways to stay active throughout your day. If you work at a desk or have to sit in front of the computer all day, set the timer on your phone or smartwatch in thirty- to forty-five-minute intervals so you will remember to get up and stretch or walk around a bit. Take a walk during your lunch hour, even if you have to walk around the parking lot at your workplace. Being sedentary all day is increasingly associated with poor health. Find ways to build more movement into your day, and watch how it will uplift your spirits!

5

Pane e Cioccolato

A Snack of Bread and Chocolate = Nostalgia

Treasured experiences are what infuse life with meaning and purpose in Italy. As an example, certain tastes, textures, and smells of food can evoke memories that bring us back to the setting, the people, and the feelings and emotions connected to that experience. This can be especially true of a childhood sweet, like chocolate, which triggers the reward centers of our brains. Dopamine, one of the neurotransmitters involved, helps turn short-term memories into long-term ones. One of my most cherished memories to this day is of the *pane e cioccolato* my grandfather would fix for himself when he came upstairs from his shoe shop to take a coffee break in the afternoon. He placed a plain chocolate bar on a piece of *sfilatino* bread, and we would talk about everything from politics to the life lessons he thought important enough for me to learn. We would write letters to send to his family in Calabria, read poetry from my pen pal in Pisa, or plan out the itinerary for our next trip to Italy—like a visit to Perugia, where I once studied at the university.

Italians love their chocolate, and Perugia is home to the largest chocolate festival in the world. It is an Etruscan town, known especially for the delicious hazelnut-crowned Baci Perugina, among other confections. My grandfather and I would not even think of discarding the silver wrappers until we read each message inscribed on them (e.g., "With your kisses I have painted my starry sky"). We would then make our way up to Venice to sit at an outdoor café along the Piazza San Marco and savor the exquisite Italian hot chocolate that has a texture more like that of pudding than warmed chocolate milk. Somehow that sojourn was all about Italian chocolate.

As gleaned from fragments of art, writings, and pottery, as early as 600 BC, chocolate was made into a beverage and used for medicinal purposes among the indigenous Mesoamerican civilizations. Italy has historically had a love affair with chocolate since it was first brought to Europe from Central America in the sixteenth century by conquistador Hernán Cortés, who in 1528 brought samples of cacao to King Charles V of Spain. Before that, Columbus, on his fourth voyage to the New World in 1502, had noticed how precious the cacao beans (which he called "almonds") were to the Mayan trading ventures.

Italian businessman and adventurer Girolamo Benzoni (1519–1572), who documented his experiences of staying in the New World for fifteen years, was one Italian who was not so enamored with the taste of chocolate. Of it, he wrote, "It seemed more like a drink for pigs than a drink for humanity... But then, as there was a shortage of wine, so as not to be always drinking water, I did like the others. The taste is somewhat bitter, it satisfies and refreshes the body, but does not inebriate, and it is the best and most expensive merchandise, according to the Indians of that country." Hardly an endorsement!

Nevertheless, chocolate continued to be in demand across Europe and Italy specifically, where chocolate was at various times discouraged by the church, coveted by nobility, or made in pharmacies. It was touted as an overall "health restorer" or as a remedy for kidney disease, digestive disorders, hemorrhoids, angina, constipation, dysentery, fatigue, dental problems, and gout—not to mention recommended as an aphrodisiac!

Italian ingenuity in creating new recipes using chocolate did not start with Pietro Ferrero (1898–1949), who, because of the shortage of chocolate following World War II, decided to try mixing whatever amount of chocolate he could obtain with the abundant supply of local hazelnuts to create

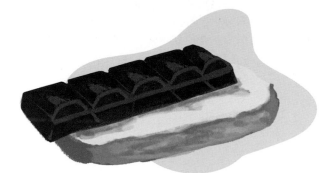

Supercrema Gianduja, later to evolve into the popular Nutella spread. Nor did it start with the trailblazing female entrepreneur (and Perugia-born clothing designer) Luisa Spagnoli, who created the Perugina chocolate factory and the hazelnut-centered Baci Perugina in 1922. Long before either Ferrero or Spagnoli was associated with innovative chocolate creations, Francesco Redi (1626–1697), physician to Cosimo III de' Medici, was experimenting with chocolate, eventually coming up with a secret jasmine-infused chocolate for the Medici court. His recipe was so coveted by nobility that it was not allowed to be revealed until after his death.

The Italian production of quality chocolate continues to be sought after throughout the world, and there are several renowned artisanal chocolate crafters across the peninsula.

Among European countries, Italy today is the seventh largest importer of cocoa beans (which must be grown within fifteen to twenty degrees of the equator) and is the second largest global exporter of chocolate (manufactured in Italy). It is also the largest global supplier of chocolate to China.

As reported in *Medical News Today*, dark chocolate, when eaten in moderation, provides antioxidants that are said to protect against heart disease, reduce inflammation and insulin resistance, and improve brain function. Because it improves blood flow to the brain, attention, memory, and verbal learning are improved in young adults, while in older adults, dark chocolate has been shown to increase cognitive function and may even be helpful in the treatment of mild cognitive impairment. Dark chocolate has also been shown to reduce negative emotions. In one study, participants were randomized to three groups and were followed for a three-week intervention period. One group consumed 85 percent dark chocolate during this period, a second group consumed 70 percent dark cocoa, and the third group served as a control, consuming no chocolate. At the end of the three weeks, only the participants in the 85 percent dark chocolate group showed a reduction in negative affect.

So what to do to satisfy your chocolate craving if you can't make it to the Eurochocolate Festival of Perugia to stroll along cobblestone streets and alleyways brimming with the scent of all things chocolate—from puzzles to personalized initials? Well, one idea is to experiment with your own chocolate-hazelnut creation, or make a pot of Italian hot chocolate at home, or invite some friends over for a jasmine-infused chocolate fondue party. And if any of that is too much to handle right now, you can just fall back on my grandfather's go-to recipe, which needs no special equipment, requires only two ingredients, and can be prepared in a flash. It is the recipe for nonno Domenico's bread and chocolate snack.

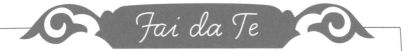

Fai da Te

PANE E CIOCCOLATO

Sometimes you might just want to enjoy the simplicity of a classic Italian dark chocolate snack. It may be an acquired taste if you have never tried it, but in the interest of keeping an open mind, I would encourage you to give it a try at least once. Savor it slowly, and you might even opt to wash it down with fragrant espresso splashed with a drop or two of sambuca.

INGREDIENTS

1 6-inch plain Italian chocolate bar, preferably Ghirardelli, Ferraro, or another Italian chocolate you can easily find at your local grocers

1 slice of thick, crusty Italian bread (homemade if you'd like to go the extra mile)

DIRECTIONS

Place the chocolate on top of the bread slice, and enjoy with a nice espresso and someone you love.

6

Le Bevande Italiane

What Italians Drink

Italy's two most popular beverages—wine and coffee—have properties that can fight depression and anxiety and, when drunk in moderation, can also make life much more pleasurable. Depression is said to affect sixteen million people in America, and about forty million people experience anxiety. As it turns out, resveratrol, a plant compound in wine, may be effective in preventing both. When it comes to *un bel caffè* (a nice cup of coffee), the research supports a potentially positive effect on mental health for this beverage too. When a Harvard neurology professor reviewed the literature on the coffee-drinking habits of over three hundred thousand people, those who drank coffee were at lower risk of depression than people who did not. One explanation for this is that it has antioxidant benefits. Coffee also has an anti-inflammatory effect that is associated with antidepressant properties.

Italians love their coffee, and Italy is the third largest coffee-consuming country overall, the United States coming in fifth. Often *una tazza di caffè espresso* (cup of espresso) is drunk while standing in a bar (in Italy, "bar" usually refers to a café bar). While the slow living movement may have its roots in the land of the dolce vita, drinking coffee is the one tradition that is still carried out at lightning speed. In two sips, an espresso is gone, and the conversation is all that lingers.

Making Italian coffee at home requires a special type of stove-top coffeepot (*moka, caffettiera napoletana, macchinetta*), which you can find online or at an Italian food store. My grandmother's *caffettiera* or *cuccumella* (or as some call it, the "*cuccuma*") is one of the most important treasures I inherited. Rich with history and imbued with memories, my Neapolitan coffeepot was old and beat up, but for many years, it filled my kitchen with the aroma of rich espresso until I had to recently switch it out for my new *moka*, which is red on top, green on the bottom, and has a silver (representing white) band across the middle, representative of the *tricolore*, the Italian flag. But while its appearance is a thing of beauty in and of itself, the real magic happens when I fill the bottom half with filtered water, then the little basket that goes inside with my fragrant Italian espresso grounds—usually Lavazza or Illy, the two most popular brands in the *bel paese*. When the water boils and drips through the grounds, the steam fills the Italian kitchen with the warmth of home.

The Italian philosophy of *non esagerare* (don't exaggerate/overdo it) applies to this daily tradition as well. Most Italians don't drink coffee nonstop throughout the day to the point of experiencing health problems or difficulty sleeping but instead may enjoy a morning cappuccino (a combination of steamed milk foam with espresso) or macchiato (espresso "marked" with a dash of steamed milk) with a fruit brioche or cornetto for breakfast (never at other times of the day, as the amount of milk is believed to impede digestion) and an espresso usually after the midday meal and/or after work.

How one drinks their *caffè* is a matter of individual preference—some like sugar, some like it with a little chocolate, some like it *amaro*, bitter or natural, or some, like in our family, preferred a *caffè corretto* ("corrected") with a splash of alcohol, such as grappa, brandy, sambuca, or anisette.

❧

Wine (vino) is the other most popular beverage in Italy. Many Italians still make their own wine or at least prefer local wine, made by others within their region. *La vendemmia*, or the grape harvest, is one of the most exciting times of year throughout Italy. It happens when summer begins to transition to the cool freshness of autumn and the white grapes, then eventually the red, are ready to be picked. Extended family and neighbors come together to harvest the grapes, make the wine, then break bread together and bask in the camaraderie.

If you want to choose an authentic Italian wine, look for the DOC or DOCG on the label to verify the authenticity. That stands for *Denominazione di origine controllata* or *Denominazione di origine controllata garantita*, which lets you know exactly what region the grapes are from. While Italians know their wines, they are not wine snobs and generally just prefer simple table wines from their own locale. Lambrusco, for example, is a fizzy red from the Emilia-Romagna region. Montepulciano is a dark, zesty wine from Abruzzo. Moscato is a sweet, sometimes fizzy wine found throughout Italy. Prosecco is a dry, frizzante white wine from Veneto.

There are two hard and fast *regole* (rules) Italians follow when it comes to coffee and wine. Italians don't drink cappuccino after 11:00 a.m. as it is considered a breakfast drink; the rest of the day, one drinks espresso. The second rule is that Italians don't drink wine to get drunk. Even though wine is consumed daily during mealtime, you rarely see a drunk Italian staggering down the street, getting rowdy, or being unable to go to work the next day because of a hangover. Breaking either one of the aforementioned rules is considered a *brutta figura* (unattractive presentation).

A few additional beverages are also synonymous with Italy's dolce vita. Especially popular in the southern regions is the famous **limoncello**, made by macerating lemon peel in alcohol. The sweetest, juiciest lemons are known to come from the Sorrento area. **Campari** is another popular drink, sold in little red glass bottles. It is a bitter, red herb-infused Italian *aperitivo* (liquor meant to stimulate appetite) that is often mixed with club soda or San Pellegrino water. Finally, **grappa**, which is made by distilling the stems, seeds, and stalks of grapes after harvesting, is used as a *digestivo* (to help digestion) after dinner. It is also an Italian folk medicine remedy for tooth-aches and other ailments.

LEARN THE VOCABULARY
OF ITALIAN CAFFÈ

Whether you decide to include coffee or wine in your diet, check first with your physician to make sure these beverages won't have a negative effect on your health. In the meantime, here are a few Italian coffee-related terms that might be fun to know:

caffè (espresso)—a small cup of very strong coffee, i.e., espresso

caffè Americano—American-style coffee but stronger; weaker than espresso and served in a large cup. It is made by diluting espresso with hot water.

caffè corretto—coffee "corrected" with a shot of grappa, cognac, or other alcohol spirit

caffè doppio—double espresso

caffè freddo—iced coffee

caffè Hag—decaffeinated coffee

caffè latte—hot milk mixed with coffee and served in a glass for breakfast *caffè macchiato*—espresso "stained" with a drop of steamed milk; small version of a cappuccino

caffè marocchino—espresso with a dash of hot milk and cocoa powder

caffè stretto—espresso with less water; rocket fuel!

cappuccino—espresso infused with steamed milk and drunk in the morning but never after lunch or dinner

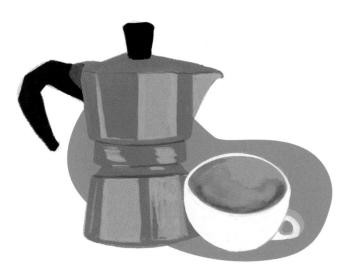

La Merenda Italiana

Italian Snack Ideas

In Pellegrino Artusi's classic 1891 Italian cookbook, he warns against snacking during the day and against the ladies "weakening their stomachs with a constant diet of sweets." (Artusi, by the way, was also the first to record a recipe for pasta and tomato sauce in the same book!) Italy has never been a country of snackers, but when its people do snack, they tend to stick to healthy choices, like fruits, vegetables, nuts, or dark chocolate. Healthy snacks like these have been associated with greater overall well-being as well as curiosity and creativity in a sample of over four hundred young adults. Studies have found that people who eat more fruits and vegetables appear to be generally happier and less depressed than people who don't eat these foods or who snack on nonnutritious foods such as chips and sweets.

While there is no paucity of studies showing the connection between healthy foods and healthy bodies, the paradigm is now beginning to shift to the connection between food and emotional well-being, life satisfaction, and happiness.

So the first dolce vita rule of snacking between meals is to **avoid it** if you are not hungry. After all, in his *Notebooks*, Leonardo da Vinci wrote that "eating contrary to inclination" (i.e., when one is not hungry) is "injurious to the health."

The second rule, if you absolutely *must* snack, however, is to choose a healthful Italian-style snack that might just satisfy—and lift your spirits too. A good example of such a *merenda della nonna* (snacks our grandmothers made) is *pane e pomodoro*. It takes about as much time as trying to open a sealed bag of processed cookies. The recipe is in the Fai da Te section below, and I hope you will give it a try.

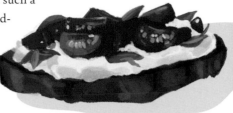

Typically, the end of a work day might call for a small snack served with an *aperitivo* meant to stimulate the appetite. The word *aperitivo* is from the Latin *aperire*, which means to "open" the stomach. The Italian version of the American happy hour was thought to have been started by distiller Antonio Benedetto Carpano, who also created one of the first types of vermouth in Turin in 1786.

Another interesting fact to consider: Italians, generally speaking, prefer **local snack ingredients** from their hometown regions. Snacks are often made fresh, using seasonal ingredients, and prepared according to family and regional tradition. In the northern Italian areas, rice and polenta are more popular, while in the south, pasta, sun-ripened tomatoes, and olive oil are staples. Similarly, coastal regions are more likely to incorporate seafood choices when planning meals and snacks. Finally, no matter what part of Italy one hails from, one can never go wrong with *pane fatto in casa* (homemade bread) as part of a healthy snack.

HOW TO ENJOY HEALTHY ITALIAN SNACKS

Here are some healthy snacks Italians might choose with their *aperitivo*. You can try them out too.

Pane e pomodoro (bread and tomato). Cut two slices of crusty bread (either homemade or purchased). Toast the bread on both sides in a hot skillet that has been lightly oiled. Slice one very ripe seasonal tomato in half, and rub each half on a slice of the toast, until the juice from the tomato soaks into the bread. Top with a clove of garlic that has been very finely chopped, a sprinkle of chopped fresh basil, and salt and pepper to taste. Finally, drizzle with just a bit of extra virgin olive oil.

Freshly picked green peas, straight from the pod. My *zia* Bettina would put these in a large basket and we would pass them around the table. So much healthier than chips or cookies!

Nuts. Italians love to snack on a handful of pistachios, walnuts, hazelnuts, or peanuts. Some experts believe that eating a few nuts now and then might even increase the feeling of happiness.

Bruschetta (pronounced broo-sketta, not bru-shetta). Brush a bit of olive oil on both sides of sliced crusty bread. Grill for a few minutes on each side. In a bowl, combine chopped ripe tomatoes, minced fresh basil, a clove of minced garlic (more if you like it), a shake or two of oregano (or some fresh minced oregano leaves), and salt and pepper to taste. Spoon over the grilled bread. Bruschetta can be made with a number of other toppings for variety. Instead of tomatoes, you can substitute mashed beans, pesto, or avocado.

Caldarroste (roasted chestnuts). Roasted chestnuts are delicious and are usually eaten around holiday time, whether slit and roasted in a frying pan, over an open fire pit, or in the oven. Italians like to add a sprinkle of salt and enjoy.

Fresh figs, nespole (loquat, or what some call the Japanese plum), or other fruit.

Fried sage leaves or zucchini flowers. Dip in a sequence of egg white and flour; then sauté in olive oil. Drain on paper towels, and sprinkle with Parmigiana Reggiano.

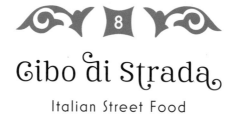

Cibo di Strada

Italian Street Food

A vibrant energy goes hand in hand with the ambiance of the Italian street food scene, where clusters of friends laugh and chat as they sample the flavors of Italy's version of outdoor fast food. Walk down the street of any major Italian city, and you will find yourself lured by the sights and smells of fast food at its finest, made with local ingredients in both traditional ways and preparations that reflect the ever-growing ethnic diversity throughout the *bel paese*. It used to be called *cibo di strada* but is now equally referred to by its fashionable English translation: street food. There is no using the drive-through and gulping down a hamburger and milkshake while driving, yet fast food is fast food, and paradoxically, despite the slower pace of Italian life, consumers are served from these kiosks without much wait time; much as they do with their *caffè*, they consume these delicacies standing up.

While the notion of Italians eating food on the fly might not make intuitive sense, there is one common denominator that remains unchanged: the social factor, which keeps loneliness and depression at bay. Small and large groups flock around kiosks, food trucks, or tiny storefronts, allowing people to come together and interact while enjoying freshly prepared foods at economical prices. Fabio Parasecoli, in an article published in *Food, Culture & Society*, points out that exciting dishes and snacks prepared by chefs combine tradition with innovative culinary offerings in the new era of Italian street food. Depending on the region, Italian street food selections will vary. Modern chefs may put their own twist on Sicilian-style arancini (rice balls), handmade pasta in containers, and pizza with fancy toppings made with special flour crusts. The foods are prepared with high-quality ingredients and are not always inexpensive.

Some Italian eateries offering street food create an atmosphere of nostalgia with specific sensory and aesthetic elements that patrons are drawn to. Pizza slices sold on the streets were popular back in the '70s when I was a young student in Perugia. I remember eating my first square of onion pizza, sans tomato sauce, and thinking I had been transported to paradise. Fried zeppole commonly appear throughout Italy's street food scenes for the feast of San Giuseppe (St. Joseph) on March 19. Simple watermelon slices and *grattachecca* (shave ice with fruit syrup) are traditional summertime street food treats, while in the winter, roasted chestnuts diffuse their nostalgic aroma on Rome's cobblestone roads around Christmastime. Often street food venues are meant to be photographed and shared on social media to market and promote as well as to highlight the experience of the social interactions.

Gusti d'Italia lists some of the most popular regional specialty street foods throughout the country:

Naples: *Frittatina di pasta*, which is a round, fried fritter made of spaghetti and stuffed with various ingredients, including provolone or mozzarella cheese and peas.

Genoa: *Farinata* is a thin pancake made of chickpea flour, water, oil, and salt

Florence: *Coccoli fritti* are little balls of fried dough sold in paper cones with prosciutto and stracchino cheese.

Palermo: *Babbalucci* are snails sautéed in onion and garlic and seasoned with pepper and parsley.

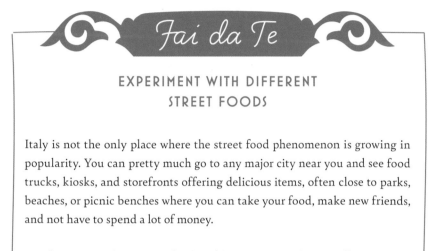

EXPERIMENT WITH DIFFERENT STREET FOODS

Italy is not the only place where the street food phenomenon is growing in popularity. You can pretty much go to any major city near you and see food trucks, kiosks, and storefronts offering delicious items, often close to parks, beaches, or picnic benches where you can take your food, make new friends, and not have to spend a lot of money.

Try doing a search on street food you'd like to try, and mark off at least one day a month to try something new. Bring a friend, or go alone and make a new friend or two.

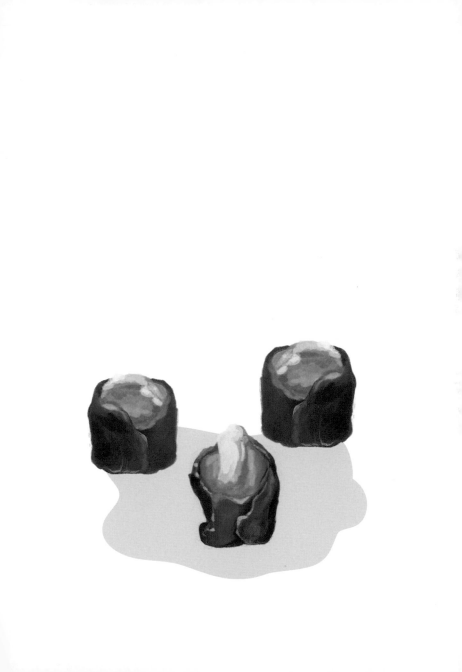

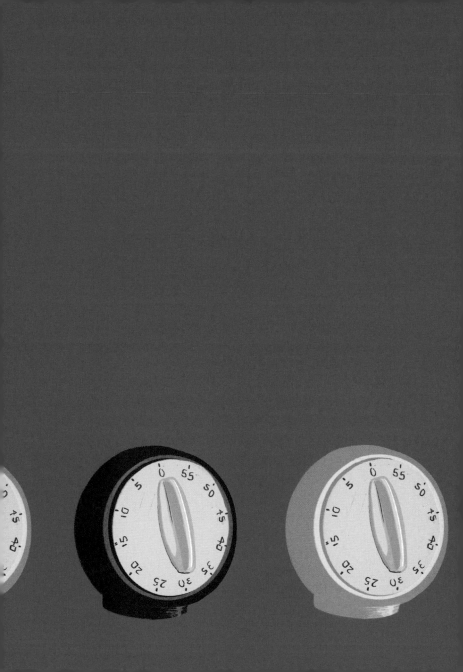

The Italian Celebration of Time

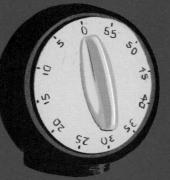
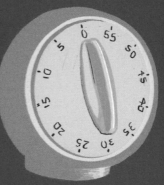

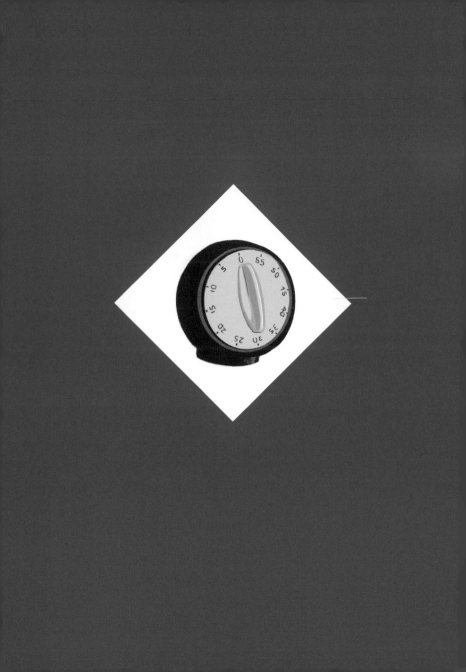

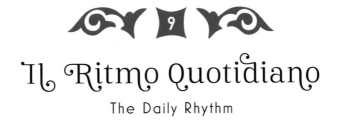

Il Ritmo Quotidiano

The Daily Rhythm

Carlo Petrini's slow food movement began in the '80s as a campaign to protest a fast-food hamburger establishment set to open near the Spanish Steps in Rome. Gradually, the movement caught on internationally and sprouted into all kinds of slow living movements and organizations, including slow cities, slow art, slow gardening, slow travel, and more. Petrini made the world aware that moving through life at breakneck speed leads to stress-related illness, exhaustion, and burnout. It robs us from fully processing the importance of our lives and the experiences at hand.

Slow cities are now sprouting up all over Italy, encouraging their residents and visitors to pause, slow down, and take note of the unique features of each locale. Slow living advocates for the protection of *intra*cultural diversity (i.e., within the country itself) by encouraging the preservation of specific traditions and traditional ways of doing things unique to that region. Traffic, noise, even crowds are limited in cities that opt to participate in the Cittaslow (slow city) movement.

The *bel paese* is also the home of slow art, proponents of which provide more relaxed tours through museums. For example, instead of rapidly eyeing artwork in succession, museumgoers view each masterpiece for fifteen minutes or so, followed by a discussion on the various nuances of each display.

Slow gardening is meant to help us strengthen our connection to the

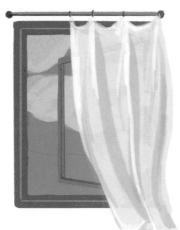

earth. It encourages good stewardship of Mother Nature and the gifts she gives us. When growing flowers or vegetables, trees or plants, those who ascribe to the slow gardening movement bring all their senses to the experience of gardening. They attend to the feel of the soil, the smell of the flowers, the sounds of watering and weeding, and the taste of the fruits and vegetables the moment they are picked. It is about gratitude for our earth and respect for the environment.

Slow living is not about being lazy or boring yourself silly by cutting your movement speed in half for no reason. To the contrary, when we slow down—just slightly below our normal pace—we eliminate excess stimulation and mental noise and are able to engage more fully with all that the present moment has to offer. We notice things we never noticed before, feel sensations we haven't felt before. A relaxing gentle calm spreads through the mind and body. "*Con calma*," Italians remind each other when they see a loved one rushing around. It means go calmly. Take it easy.

Living at a slower, more conscious pace forces us to think about what we are doing and fully engage in our lives. We discover new things about ourselves when we put an end to perfunctory robotic living.

Italians have ascribed to slower-paced living long before the official slow food movement came about in the '80s. Whenever I go to Italy, I can't help but be aware of how the days seem to dawdle instead of race by, despite the same twenty-four hours in a day. I rarely ask myself "Where did the day go?" because I am immersed in every moment, with none taken for granted.

The Stoic philosopher Seneca the Younger, in his treatise *On the Shortness of Life*, warned against wasting the time we have on the earth in "laborious dedication to useless tasks." Doing this, he warned, makes life fly by, leaving us feeling empty when we reach the end and wishing we had more experiences that were meaningful to us. He wrote, "The greatest obstacle to living is *expectancy*, which hangs on tomorrow and loses today."

Italians are not in a hurry. Quality living takes priority over rushed living, a fact evident throughout history. It takes roughly 250 hours to hand-craft a violin, first invented in the sixteenth century by Andrea Amati of Cremona, Italy. Michelangelo dedicated two years of continuous and careful work to sculpt his masterpiece, *David*. Dante dedicated twelve years of his life to writing the narrative poem *The Divine Comedy*. Filippo Brunelleschi built the largest dome in the world in the span of sixteen years—Santa Maria del Fiore, which stands out in Florence as a breathtaking architectural treasure that seems to defy gravity. Brunelleschi had no formal architectural training in 1418 when he won the bid to build the Duomo. He simply took all the time he needed to come up with innovative ways to structure it without the traditional central supports or buttresses commonly used to support the weight of domes in that period. Similarly, traditional balsamic vinegar in Modena is aged for twenty-five years as certain grapes are crushed, their liquid boiled over an open flame, then transferred over the years to barrels of various woods that impart their own flavor to the exquisite final product.

A quality life affords you just the right amount of unhurried time to achieve pride and satisfaction in whatever you apply yourself to. Here are some ideas to get you off the fast train and onto the slow boat to more joy.

Fai da Te

TAKING LIFE AT A SLOWER PACE

Slowing down a bit, instead of rushing through your day, helps to make you more aware of the details that bring happiness and pleasure to your life. It helps you to notice what you would normally gloss over. Here are some ways to enjoy a more relaxed approach to living.

❀ Make a recipe that involves a bit more time to prepare than usual or a long cooking time, such as old-fashioned rice or oats instead of instant. Try percolating coffee instead of using a drip machine. Make cookies or a pie by hand, including the crust, instead of buying one at the bakery.

❀ Approach housework at a slightly slower pace than you usually do, letting yourself experience the satisfaction of cleaning each item thoroughly as you go along. When I was young, we had a summer cottage on the shore with a black-and-brown tile floor. At the beginning of each season, I would wash and then wax the floors on my hands and knees with rags. I felt so proud of getting each dark square of the floor to shine like a mirror when I was done.

❀ Take sixty seconds to just close your eyes and meditate several times throughout the day.

❀ Spend more time doing what you love, slightly less time on your obligatory to-do list.

❀ Allow yourself to relax when you feel tired instead of pushing yourself to keep going.

Il Dolce Far Niente

The Sweetness of Doing Nothing

There is a scene in the movie *Eat Pray Love* where the protagonist is sitting in a local barbershop in Italy while her language tutor and his friend get their hair cut. The two men, along with the barber, are trying to explain the meaning of the Italian phrase *il dolce far niente*, the sweetness of doing nothing. They begin a lively conversation, musing about how Americans seem to need permission to enjoy the feeling of taking a break from the rat race of routine. They presume they should have to earn it or be told that they deserve a break today. Italians, on the other hand, *know* they deserve breaks, but for them, it doesn't mean plopping in front of the TV with a beer for the evening. It means taking a moment to reflect or a whole day to enjoy carefree time with good friends, just for the joy of it.

Roman emperor Marcus Aurelius believed that retreating into oneself provides immediate and perfect tranquility. And "tranquility," he wrote, "is nothing else than the good ordering of the mind."

When was the last time *you* opted out of the daily rat race and carved out an hour or so of your day to do absolutely nothing but relax, regroup, and reconnect to who you really are without letting social media, the nightly news, magazine images, or the judgment of coworkers, family, and friends put limits on your creativity? When every waking moment is used up rushing from one assignment to another, you rob yourself of what Abraham Maslow referred to as *peak experiences*, those life-changing moments of insight that lead to personal transformation. You can't achieve these when your thoughts are cluttered, worried, disorganized, or entirely goal-focused.

I once spent an entire afternoon just observing life at an outdoor café on the Piazza San Marco in Venice. Observation was the process that fueled the creativity of Leonardo da Vinci, and it is easy to understand why. All around me, I drank in a collage of sights, sounds, and smells of pigeons flapping about, Italians embracing as if they hadn't seen each other in years, peaceful protesters carrying signs, and tourists from all over the world snapping photos from every angle of the diverse combination of architectural styles contained in the splendor of the Basilica of San Marco. Immersing myself in the present experience brings my mind to a place of serenity, gives me clarity, and helps me savor the moments of life that can only be experienced once.

Il dolce far niente is about making the time to unwind without guilt, banishing shoulds, musts, or worries, and using your heightened senses to fully experience the moments that will never return again. The next time you stand at the edge of a riverbank, delight in the trickle of the water flow! The next time you hike up a mountain, drink in the expansiveness of Mother Nature's panorama. A friend from Napoli revealed that after work every day, instead of going directly into the house, he goes straight to garden for an hour or so before dinner to unwind. While he's watering and weeding, the day's cares and worries melt away before he heads back in the house for dinner.

Planning a daily block of time each day for simply "being" is as important as the time you plan for tasks and responsibilities—perhaps even more. A tourist once asked a native resident of Amalfi who was sunning himself, "What do you do?" The man sunning himself looked puzzled at the question and then answered, "*This* is what I do!"

Of course, you don't necessarily have to watch clouds roll across the sky or waves crash against the shore. You can design your downtime in any way that makes you feel relaxed and recharged. *Il dolce far niente* is the Italian antidote to stress. If you are not used to allowing yourself the luxury of carving out a block of time to experience the sweetness of doing nothing (in particular), now is the time, and here are some ideas to which you will certainly want to add your own.

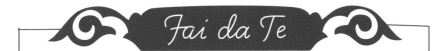

Fai da Te

HOW TO PRACTICE *IL DOLCE FAR NIENTE*

You don't need an exotic and costly vacation to de-stress and recharge your energy. Brief periods of *il dolce far niente* are built into the fabric of Italian life. Here are some simple ways you too can take a periodic break from the monotony of routine, the stress of deadlines, and overall hurried living.

❀ Turn off the TV and sign off from social media and your electronic devices for fifteen minutes while you close your eyes, sit back, and take a few slow, deep breaths. I like to count to four as I inhale through the nose, hold the breath for four, then exhale slowly through pursed lips to another slow count of four.

❀ Get outside and *observe*. Watch the bees flitting across the flowers. Let your worries melt away as you take in the neighbor's laundry dancing in the breeze. Be aware of the hum of a distant lawn mower, the drone of an overhead plane, or the playful song of a bird.

- ✿ Sip your early-morning or evening beverage in a spot where you can see how the sunrise or sunset colors the sky. In coastal Italian towns, communities come together in awe before the sun sets over the water.

- ✿ Go fishing off the end of a pier, or sit at the end of the pier and let the sound and sight of the moving waters send you into a trancelike state.

- ✿ Drift around on a pool float in a calm body of water or a pool.

- ✿ Through a good pair of headphones, listen to soft instrumental music.

- ✿ Slowly savor the taste, sight, and smell of every bite of an apple, every sip of wine, every bite of chocolate you consume.

- ✿ Color, paint, or draw freestyle.

- ✿ Take a nap.

- ✿ Write a poem or song.

- ✿ Experiment with a musical instrument.

- ✿ Chill out on a park bench and people-watch.

- ✿ Walk barefoot along the beach or in the grass.

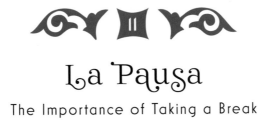

La Pausa

The Importance of Taking a Break

While some might need a reminder that a regular break from routine is a good thing, refreshing changes of pace have been woven into the fabric of Italian life for centuries. The following examples prove my point.

The word *siesta* comes from the Latin word *sexta*, referring to the sixth hour of daylight. The ancient Romans went home for lunch during siesta (or *riposo*) and then would either nap or relax with family or friends for a couple of hours. Today, especially in the smaller southern Italian towns (and to a lesser extent in the north), mom-and-pop shops, banks, pharmacies, and restaurants close their doors and lower their street-level *saracinesca* (rolling shutters), and workers still go home in the middle of the afternoon. They may enjoy a home-cooked meal and afterward a walk or perhaps a short nap before returning to work. The siesta serves to slow the daily rhythm and refresh the body and mind.

Ferragosto is another way Italians take a pause from the daily grind by leaving the hot city behind for a week or two around the time of the Catholic Feast of the Assumption, the day the Virgin Mary left the earth and ascended into heaven. *Ferragosto* (originally *Feriae Augusti*) originated with the Roman emperor Augustus in 18 BC. Although the holiday is formally recognized on August 15, the mass exodus from busy Italian cities to the shoreline or mountains often comes a week or two earlier. Italian highway operators often discourage drivers from traveling on August 8, using the *bollino nero* (a black traffic sign), which refers to the worst traffic day of the year.

Un pisolino (a nap) is a common Italian luxury and requires no special getaway to indulge. A comfortable snooze on a chaise longue at the beach or under a shady tree in the spring breeze is believed to be as important to the body as exercise. According to the National Sleep Foundation, napping can enhance performance and reduce mistakes and accidents. Napping also has psychological as well as physical benefits.

Fare il ponte literally translates as "to make the bridge," but in Italy, when someone prepares to *fare il ponte*, they are planning to take a long weekend, typically in conjunction with a national holiday that falls in the middle of the week, but not necessarily.

La notte bianca (white night) happens in cities all over Italy. It is a night when lights stay on and people stay awake from sunset to sunrise to revel in Italian culture. Fashion and food are highlighted. Museums and shops stay open, and streets are filled with music and entertainment. It is a break from the same old routine and a time for people to come together to enjoy merriment and to party like an Etruscan. As one character in Verdi's *Attila* says, "You many have the universe if I may have Italy." The excitement of a sleepless nightlong Italian celebration convinces me he was right.

Fai da Te

HOW TO TAKE A BREAK FROM ROUTINE

Breaking with routine, whether just after a midday meal or for a change of scenery, can increase our quality of life. In one study of over one thousand participants in Denmark, researchers found that taking a break from the regular use of social media increased both well-being and positive emotions in those who took a time-out from Facebook for a while, versus those in the control group who continued to be regularly engaged in that platform.

* If you work in an office, resist eating lunch at your desk while continuing to work. Take your lunch outside if the weather is nice, and find a pleasant area to eat. Take a leisurely stroll afterward. Before you begin to work again, take a minute or so at your desk to close your eyes and do a five-minute meditation. It will refresh you with new energy to face the rest of your day.

* If you are home during the day, schedule your activities around the time you have blocked out for your *riposo*. Make a healthy lunch for yourself, and invite family, friends, or neighbors to share it with you. Set the table beautifully; perhaps add a vase of fresh flowers from the garden or a flowering plant. After lunch, set aside some time to meditate, read an inspirational passage, or take a quick nap before getting on with the rest of your day. Incorporating the Italian tradition of *siesta* as part of your lifestyle is a way to make yourself a priority and reclaim your energy and passion for life.

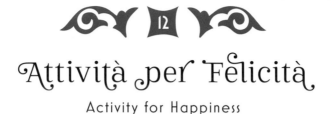

Attività per Felicità

Activity for Happiness

If you ask Italians on the street what they do for exercise, you are bound to get as many answers as Italy has regions. Many have fun participating in (in addition to watching) sports and are especially passionate about *calcio* (soccer). Enthusiasm for one's favorite team (Juventus, Milan, etc.) spills over into daily life, and you will see friends of all ages scrimmaging or starting up an impromptu game in little piazzas and parks right in their neighborhood. Other sports commonly practiced among Italians for both fitness and fun include basketball, volleyball, swimming, bicycling, hiking, and almost any other activity that takes them out into the fresh air and provides a way to share good times with friends.

The ancient Romans realized that regular physical activity was indispensable for staying strong and in shape. Roman bathhouses included an open-air exercise area, called the palaestra, surrounded by colonnades. While some trained heavily for sport, the thinking then, as today, was that *moderate* physical activity made the most sense. According to the research, both unstructured physical activity as well as programmed exercise routines can make us feel more confident and happier and can even increase our sense of self-worth. Staying active can also sharpen our mental performance and reduce stress, anxiety, and depression.

The ancient Roman philosopher Seneca the Younger, in one of his

Letters (XV), wrote that some exercises, like running, jumping, and brandishing weights, are "plain and easy" yet tire the body quickly, so it is important to do them quickly, then come back to exercising the mind. Italy has not changed its stance on the importance of

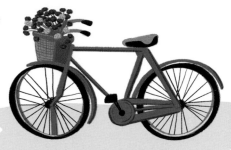

staying active while at the same time avoiding overdoing it.

Many Italian women, like Sophia Loren, for instance, stay in shape by doing gentle calisthenics. In her book *Women and Beauty*, this ageless beauty admitted that while she takes exercising very seriously, you will not find her doing frenzied, heart-stopping, pavement-pounding routines. She feels that jogging is not the best exercise for the joints, and to add to that, the air pollution is harmful to one's lungs.

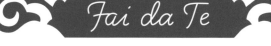

Fai da Te

ITALIAN-STYLE EXERCISE

Italians generally take a moderate but consistent approach to exercise—such as walking or even just staying active throughout the day. Here are some ways that you can incorporate some dolce vita fitness routines in your own life.

Seek (don't avoid) stairs. If you live along the Amalfi Coast, it is easy to climb stairs, since the villages are built into the side of mountainous terrain. If you want to go anywhere on the Amalfi

Coast, you have to scale steep steps going up and down to your home, and I have seen countless elders do this with more vim and vigor than much younger tourists are able to muster. I can't imagine those living in Amalfi, Praiano, or Atrani needing to work out on an exercise stair stepper!

Don't stay seated. Shepherds in Sardinia walk all day, and that is one reason there is a high rate of residents who live to one hundred or beyond. The lesson here is that all-day movement is good. In fact, being sedentary is now considered by researchers to be as dangerous to your health as smoking. My paternal family lives on a farm about an hour and a half from Naples. Their days from sunrise to sunset are composed of physical work. Farm life requires cleaning animal stalls, planting and harvesting crops, and making most food from scratch the way my grandmother did when she grew up there. Nevertheless, the joy of productive physical work is second only to the health benefits you reap by staying active.

Go for a bike ride. When I was staying in Parma while conducting body image research, I would open the wooden shutters early in the morning to let the sunshine flood my room, only to be enchanted by the sight of beautiful, well-dressed older women on their way home from the open-air market on bicycles with two grocery bags either hooked over the handlebars or tucked into a basket over the front wheel. Biking is a wonderful form of transportation that, in addition to being fun, also provides you with the cognitive and physical benefits of staying active.

Take a walk. Because it is so difficult to park in the larger cities, Italians walk (or bike) to most of their local destinations. Whenever

I am in Rome, as in many of the cities and smaller towns throughout Italy, I stroll through the Piazza Navona or other main avenues
and witness the nationally practiced early-evening promenade, or
passeggiata, whereby the whole family gets out to walk, socialize,
or window-shop. This common ritual is the antithesis to the couch
potato syndrome that is so easy to slip into!

Take an active vacation. When Italians go on vacation, they often
choose fun sporting activities, like camping and hiking through
the woods, swimming in the crystal-blue waters surrounding the
peninsula, or skiing down the trails of the Apennine or Dolomite
mountains. They don't need a smartphone app that has them chasing down cartoon shapes to get them outdoors and moving.

Dance! The characteristic Italian tarantella is not only great exercise, it is a great pathway to emotional and physical healing too,
according to Dr. Alessandra Belloni, the international authority
on this dance form. For one thing, certainly breaking a sweat from
such a fun activity cleanses your pores as well as burns calories, but
you cannot possibly feel depressed when you are rapidly dancing
to the lively, upbeat rhythm of the "spider dance." I keep a couple
of tarantella music selections on my playlist so I can take activity bursts throughout the day when I'm at the office. Just getting
up and dancing for even a few minutes clears the head and keeps
your body responsive to regular activity. When you move intermit-
tently throughout the day, you can change your mood as you stay
in shape. Dancing has been shown to lower depression and promote
well-being, no matter what type of dancing you prefer.

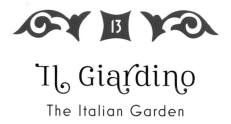

Il Giardino

The Italian Garden

Around 42 percent of Italians have gardens, and gardening is one of the most popular activities in the *bel paese*, especially among families. There is no paucity of research confirming the effects of gardening on happiness and well-being. The benefits of interacting with nature include the satisfaction derived from purposeful activity, an opportunity to be creative, and a way to express our nurturing needs as we get older to make up for the inevitable losses we experience.

Tending to a traditional Italian vegetable garden provides physical activity, makes the body feel fantastic, and calms the mind. Italians will tell you that despite the hard work that gardening requires, working with the earth is a passion and a joy. Some have said they spend as much time in their gardens as they do caring for their children. As the old Italian saying goes, "*L'orto vuole un uomo morto*"— "It takes a dead man to grow a vegetable garden." In other words, planting, watering, and weeding require such a commitment of time that you really can't walk away from it.

Gardening in some form is a widespread part of Italian life. I "apprenticed" in my grandparents' Italian gardens year after year. I watched my grandfather prepare the soil, anticipating the moment he would signal me to sprinkle in the vegetable seeds or place the little tomato plants into their grooves when the shoots had to be separated. Then my grandmother and I would tend to her flowers, which gave our modest inner-city home a sense of Italian beauty and majesty. We would weed the irises and tulips that lined our tiny backyard, water the hydrangeas, and prune the rose bushes that bordered the front wall. My other grandparents—the ones who emigrated to the United States from a small farming village in Italy—also knew how to cultivate every inch of their backyard and then some. To them, grass-covered lawns were a waste of space when you could grow your own food and be self-sufficient all year long. We hoisted water up from a bucket in a well to moisten the soil around their grape arbor, and before the harsh New England winter, they would insulate, wrap, and bury their fig trees, which started from a twig from their motherland.

For Italians, gardening is no trivial pursuit. It is a way of life. It is a way of staying active and nourishing the body correctly. It is also a way of sharing the gifts of one's labor with neighbors. Gardening is a way for generations to work together with a common goal. My father and his brothers would make wine from the grapes in their grape arbor. Grandmother made grape jelly with what was left over. From the tomatoes, basil, and garlic, she made pasta sauce and canned it to be enjoyed throughout the winter. She pickled the eggplant, peppers, cauliflower, and zucchini, dried the oregano, and preserved the beans to enjoy with pasta for a delicious supper on a cold winter's night. Seeds collected from the overripe plants were washed, dried, and saved for the next planting season. Compost was made from table scraps and garden debris. Everything was sustainable and organic. Italy is one of the largest agricultural producers in the European Union.

In addition to yielding beautiful flowers and essential produce, some Italian gardens are created only to provide visual beauty. In Renaissance times among the wealthy classes, summer villa gardens were ornate and architecturally designed to provide solace, meditation, and a respite from busy, hot urban life. Imagine water fountains, grottoes, statues, structured hedge mazes, and perhaps as a focal point a pond equipped with a couple of rowboats, where one could drift into cerebral tranquility. There might be a garden section with fruits or medicinal herbs, but mainly the garden was a natural work of art.

No matter how small the growing space may be, Italians will combine the aesthetics of flowers with the utility of fruits and vegetables. You might catch sight of a little bench or seating area under the shady grape arbor from which one can water, or a holy shrine devoted to St. Francis or the Blessed Mother Mary. For those who live in city apartments, you will see colorful pots filled with growing herbs like parsley, basil, rosemary, and oregano and rich red cherry tomatoes along the edges of the balcony.

Gardening has been shown to positively impact both emotional and physical health of those who plant, water, reap, and admire. Ecopsychologists say some of the benefits of gardening include the following:

❉ Aesthetic beauty that lifts our mood

❉ A connection with nature, which affirms our place in the universe

❉ Physical exercise from bending, weeding, hoeing, and digging

❉ Fresh air and vitamin D from the sunshine

❉ A sense of achievement

❉ A meditation effect as we work with the soil

❉ Stress reduction as we immerse ourselves in the process

❉ Engagement with life

❉ Greater consumption of fruits and vegetables

❉ Foods to feed your body and flowers to feed your soul

Fai da Te

START YOUR OWN ITALIAN GARDEN

Gardening can be a source of pleasure and satisfaction. It is also a great way to squeeze some physical activity into your day and enjoy some uplifting fresh air and sunshine. Start out small, whether planting beautiful flowers or colorful vegetables.

If you are new to gardening or want to go back to the basics, start by finding a book on how to start a vegetable garden or, if you don't have a garden space, how to grow vegetables in pots and containers. There are also plenty of free resources on the internet, which include videos that show you step by step how to grow a garden organically, so you don't have to use any kinds of pesticides. While you can't bring the _bel paese_ soil or climate to your backyard, you can easily find classic Italian heirloom seeds to start with in online stores such as the following: seedsofitaly.com, growitalian.com, theheirloomseedstore.com, and amazon.com.

Remember to let a few plants go to seed; then collect, wash, dry, and store the seeds so you won't have to keep repurchasing them.

Don't forget to designate a little sitting area from which you can water your plants and enjoy the sights, smells, and sounds of nature responding to all your efforts. A garden, no matter how big or how small, can be a meditative sanctuary that feeds your soul as much as it refreshes your body.

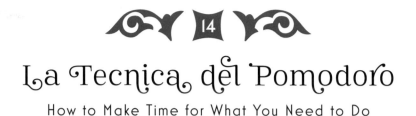

La Tecnica del Pomodoro

How to Make Time for What You Need to Do

When Francesco Cirillo was a student at Guido Carli International University in the early 1990s, he realized he was wasting time with too many distractions and learning very little. He had trouble focusing and accomplishing his study goals, until one day he took a kitchen timer shaped like a tomato (*pomodoro*) and challenged himself to work for just ten minutes straight without interruption. One thing led to another, and the Pomodoro Technique was born. The idea became so popular that he developed it further, wrote a book about it, and gave workshops to entrepreneurs and others who needed a simple way to manage their time, become more efficient at accomplishing their goals, and have time left over for other interests.

Whether you have tasks that you have been putting off, projects that you don't particularly like doing but must be done, or goals that you want to accomplish but find yourself getting lost in a sea of distractions, the Pomodoro Technique might be just what you need to be more productive. Using time management techniques not only helps you gain momentum with respect to getting things done, but gaining control over your time will help you feel less stressed, as was found in a study that examined stress levels in academic students before and after time management training. Today, with all the distractions of social media, smartphones dinging with instant message alerts, Netflix, YouTube, and television news, it is easy to get off course and find

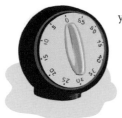

yourself disappointed at the end of the day because you didn't accomplish what you had intentions of doing. The act of setting a mechanical timer and placing check marks on a piece of paper marking off the completion of mini steps along the way will increase your chances of attaining your intended goal.

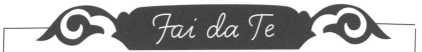

Fai da Te

MANAGE YOUR TIME, ITALIAN STYLE

You can find out more on the author's website, FrancescoCirillo.com/pomodoro-technique, but for a condensed, perhaps oversimplified version, you can start using these steps.

1 Decide what task you would like to get done.

2 Gather a mechanical timer (or use the timer on your smartphone), paper, and a pencil.

3 Set the timer for twenty-five minutes, and make a pact with yourself to stay focused for that block of time. Make a check mark on the paper for having completed that time on task. Take a five- to ten-minute break when the timer goes off.

4 Set the timer for three more blocks of time (twenty-five minutes each), and after each one, take the same short break, and put another check mark on the paper.

5 After the fourth twenty-five-minute block of time, take a longer break of twenty-five to thirty minutes. If more time is needed to complete your project, repeat the entire process.

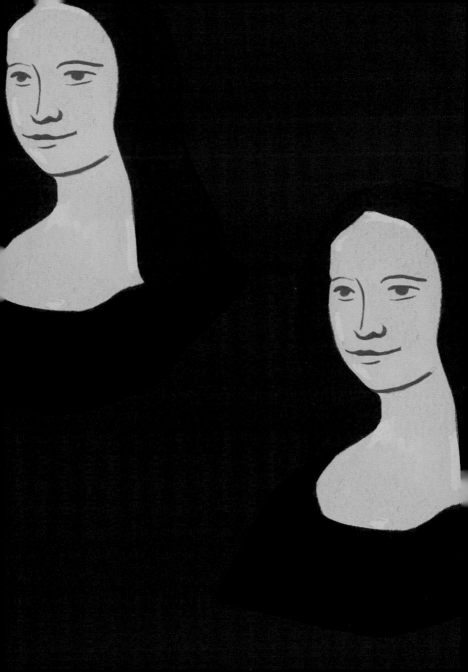

The Italian Celebration of Self

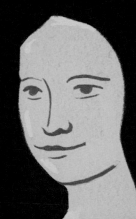

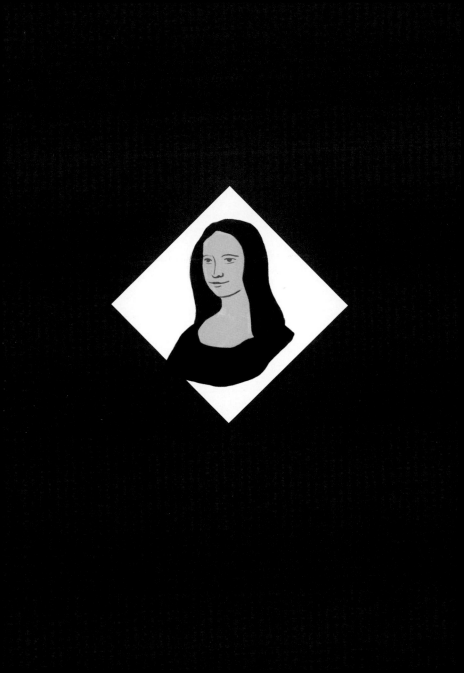

Il Sorriso Italiano

The Italian Smile

Venetian-born Pope John Paul I (1912–1978) had the shortest reign in papal history; he died thirty-three days after his inauguration in Vatican City. But he still had quite an impact in that short amount of time. He shunned the pomp and circumstance of his position, preferring instead to connect with and serve the people. He was the first pope who refused to be crowned, and he tried (unsuccessfully) to resist the practice of *la sedia gestatoria* (the practice of carrying the pope on a raised chair in order to let the public have a better view as he moved through the crowds). All popes who succeeded him instead used the popemobile. In his brief role as the pontiff, there is one thing people still remember about him today: his *sorriso* (smile). It was unforgettable, as he was rarely seen without it. That warm smile made Italians feel close to him, as if he were more a family member than a high-level Catholic authority. His Holiness is still known today as "the smiling pope," who was so loved, perhaps because he knew that "a cheerful look brings joy to the heart" (Proverbs 15:30).

Guillaume Duchenne (1806–1875) was a French neurologist most noted for his research that made a distinction between a sincere smile (referred to as the Duchenne smile), involving contractions of the muscles surrounding both the mouth and the eyes, and a more intentional or polite smile, involving movement of the mouth only. The former is a smile of enjoyment, the latter a smile of obligation. A sincere smile is more welcoming, more quickly recognized, and it makes people feel more of a connection with the smiler. But beyond improving one's social life, a *genuine* smile can do much more.

Smiling makes us feel good. Both Charles Darwin and William James believed that our outward facial expressions could alter or intensify our inward emotions. This is called the facial feedback hypothesis. In other words, the mere *act* of smiling can actually elevate mood, and a sustained positive mood over time can even extend life, as was found in one study of rural Italians aged 90 to 101. Their longevity, despite age-related physical decline, was associated with confidence in overcoming adversity with a positive attitude. Examples of the participants' comments included "I am always thinking of the best. There is always a solution in life"; "Life is what it is and must be faced...always!"; "I am always ready for changes. I think changes bring life and give chances to grow."

Some smiles leave us curious, as they seem to hold a secret. One such smile that has been studied for over five hundred years is the mysteriously intriguing smile of Leonardo da Vinci's *Mona Lisa*. Harvard scientists have tried to understand why, when looking at the painting, we sometimes see a distinct smile and sometimes not. Leonardo combined painstaking skill and meticulous detail when casting shadows in his artwork. It turns out that *Mona Lisa*'s smile looks more defined when observing it through our peripheral vision, which has fewer photoreceptors and is thus more adept at seeing shadows, like the one cast by the subject's cheekbones. On the other hand, we perceive more ambiguity in her smile when we are looking at it straight on using our foveal vision (the area at the back of the retina that contains the highest number of light receptors). Other researchers, who have ever so subtly manipulated the corners of the *Mona Lisa*'s mouth, found that observers rate her original smile as a happier expression than any of the manipulated variations. *Mona Lisa*'s smile is undeniably magnetic.

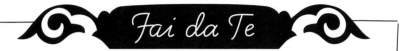

Fai da Te

SMILE MORE

My advice here is quite simple yet can make a huge difference in your life: smile every chance you get. Even when you don't feel like it. Smiling, in addition to making others want to be around you, can actually improve your mood. When negative emotions get the better of you, put on a smile, even if you have to force yourself. Keep that smile there for a full minute or longer, and note how the negative energy dissipates and that smile becomes genuine.

La Sprezzatura

Making the Difficult Look Easy

Despite all his vocal training and hard work keeping his singing voice in tip-top form, despite the nerves that always got to him in his first few seconds onstage (as he described in an interview with Larry King), Frank Sinatra, who was born to Italian immigrants, always managed to look smooth and cool and delivered his songs perfectly and effortlessly. Cognitive psychologists call this phenomenon "automaticity," where, with a lot of hard work and practice, you become so proficient at a particular skill that you can practically do something else at the same time and never miss a beat. In his 1528 *The Book of the Courtier*, Baldassare Castiglione referred to this concept as *sprezzatura*, or the art of making the difficult look easy. Sinatra appeared smooth and confident as he romanced his audiences with the expressiveness of those ocean-blue eyes and laid-back gestures. The songs he sang were no longer about a studied amount of resonance or the shaping of vowels (e.g., the sound of "ah" that he warned should always be sung as "uh"), but now it was the heartfelt lyrics, the telling of a story, that transported his fans away from their everyday cares to another world.

Sprezzatura. Italian actor Marcello Mastroianni had it. Fiat CEO Gianni Agnelli had it. But Sophia Loren was also a shining example. They were smooth, they were suave, they had impeccable style, carried themselves with grace, and were so good at what they did as to make even complex tasks seem easy to onlookers.

Castiglione essentially laid out a template for manners and civility pertaining to the "ideal" gentleman of the royal courts. While his philosophy was primarily targeted to the art of being a gentleman, he also added advice on proper womanliness. Admittedly the book was written when times were much different, but the universal takeaway is simply a recipe for how to acquire a charismatic personality.

By most definitions, charisma is defined as a compelling attractiveness or charm that elicits the admiration—even the devotion—of others. We associate charisma with qualities of likeability, leadership, confidence, and competence. We find it hard not to admire those who exhibit such traits.

Renowned Italian physicist Enrico Fermi displayed these traits as described by the late MIT professor Bernard Feld, once a graduate assistant of Fermi, in reminiscing about watching his mentor at the lectern. In the postwar era in a town near Como, Fermi delivered a series of lectures on the physics of pions and nucleons. In Dr. Feld's recollection, "Fermi was at the height of his powers; bringing order and simplicity out of confusion, finding connections between seemingly unrelated phenomena; wit and wisdom emerging from lips white as usual, from contact with chalk; in that clear, resonant voice that never lost the soft Italian vowel endings on a perfectly colloquial American delivery."

Feld was describing a riveting lecturer who knew how to inspire students, making them want to emulate him and unravel the complexity of even the most difficult scientific principles. Compare this to a time as a student when you may have fallen into an academic coma at having to sit through a lecture delivered in a dry monotone by someone reading from pages of notes.

Sprezzatura is not just about developing skills, which although practiced with great effort in private, could be executed with ease and effortlessness in public. It is also about acquiring knowledge across different areas, such as music, literature, and art, so as to be interesting and conversant, thus creating an Italian art form of one's public persona.

One who exhibits sprezzatura displays civility and impeccable manners.

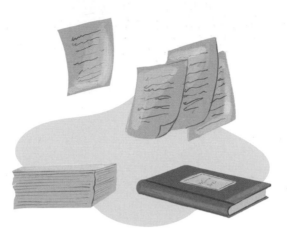

It might be the young person who gives up their seat for an elder or a man who opens a car door for a woman. Helpfulness and chivalry with a smile are what I remember of a boy whom I will call Marco, who came to America to live with his grandparents at the age of sixteen. Our families were close; in fact they were *compaesani* from the old country. When we all got together for dinner, Marco took such delight in helping serve! An expression of satisfaction took over his face as he set each plate in front of us, making sure we had our napkins at hand, asking with heartfelt attentiveness if we needed anything else. He made each of us around the table feel like a royal guest with focused attention. The image of Marco's confidence and generosity of spirit was a people magnet. Who isn't drawn to someone who can make excellence look effortless? Who isn't inspired by such an example to go out and be the best he or she can be too?

Sprezzatura is an attractive quality. Getting really proficient at something can also lead to a better social life, because people want to be around those with confidence, self-assurance, and accomplishment. Most important, self-efficacy (a belief in your capacity to succeed at your objectives) has been associated with greater happiness and greater overall life satisfaction. Here is one way to start.

Fai da Te

ACQUIRE SPREZZATURA

If you don't have at least one skill you can practically perform with your eyes closed, here are some tips to increase your SQ (sprezzatura quotient) and also your self-confidence:

❁ Choose an attainable yet challenging skill you think you'd enjoy. It can be reconnecting with an instrument you used to play years ago, learning a new language, or perfecting a recipe handed down from your grandmother.

❁ Make some progress on it every day by practicing, inching closer and closer to being able to do it effortlessly.

❁ Get expert instruction or the materials you need to teach yourself to take you to the next level.

❁ Find someone to emulate, as an example to aspire to.

❁ Don't let minor flops discourage you; instead glitches can become the fuel you need to be more determined than ever to improve.

❁ Whether you are an artisan, scientist, homemaker, or sandwich vendor, achieving mastery is an important value in the Italian culture, and it can be a powerful tool for living la dolce vita. All you need do is practice, practice, practice. Then share your skill with the world.

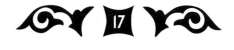

Le Parole

The Power of Words to Cultivate Serenity

The Roman Stoics believed that the key to a happy life lies in the ability to control our mental state, since we have little control over external forces. Loved ones pass away. The horrors broadcast on the news frighten us. We fall ill. A family member cuts us out of their life, leaving us confused, angry, or hurt.

Italian psychiatrist Roberto Assagioli (1888–1974, author of *Act of Will*) understood this well. He himself was no stranger to human suffering. He was jailed for being a pacifist by Mussolini's Fascist regime, persecuted by the Nazis, forced into hiding with his family, and faced unbearable grief after the death of his only son. Despite such adversity, he left a legacy of psychosynthesis (*psicosintesi*), a psychospiritual model of human development that emphasizes the positive side of human nature. A contemporary of both Freud and Jung, Assagioli, while embracing some of the elements of his colleagues' theories, took psychology in a more holistic direction, incorporating the mental, physical, emotional, and spiritual aspects of an individual. He strongly believed in our conscious ability to make meaningful changes to our lives as opposed to being helplessly driven at the hands of our unconscious instinct (as in Freud's psychoanalytic theory). Psychosynthesis emphasizes our potential to grow and evolve throughout our lives.

Outside the context of psychotherapy, Assagioli also envisioned his practical techniques to have applications in the areas of personal, educational, community, and social settings. I would like to share with you a few of his techniques for mental well-being. Although not a substitute for psychotherapy when needed, these self-help applications are simple and effective.

The technique of evocative words. Dr. Assagioli believed that certain words, like *joy, serenity, courage*, etc., have an ability to affect our state of mind, our physical state, and the acts that correspond to the words. Just seeing and reflecting on these words reinforces their effectiveness and activates the quality that the words signify. The procedure is this: First, choose a word that expresses a feeling or quality you want to develop in yourself. It could be the word *appreciation, friendship, calm, serenity, tenacity, wonder*, etc. We will take the word *joy* as an example. Write the word *joy* down on several note cards, and place them throughout your house where you will see them, perhaps on your nightstand, desk, or on a wall. Next, in a state of relaxation, focus on that word for a minute or two. You can repeat it to yourself, contemplate its meaning, and feel yourself absorbing it.

The technique of substitution. Dr. Assagioli was convinced that when attention is centered on a certain object, it gives that object energy and makes it more salient in our awareness. When we focus on unwanted thoughts or images, negative energy is drawn to us like a magnet and produces a negative mood. Using what he called our "skillful will," we can displace one image for another. We can direct ourselves to look at, hear, or read uplifting materials that give us joy. Substitution helps to take our focus away from negativity.

The "acting as if" technique. This means acting as if you are already joyful (even if you are not feeling joy at the moment). We can only exert limited control over our internal feelings and emotions but can more easily impact our mood by first directing our external actions. We can actually begin to change how we feel when we use our bodies according to the feeling we want to produce. For example, when we feel upset or angry about something minor, we can use joyful facial expressions, put on some music and dance, or have a cheerful conversation with someone.

According to those who knew him, whether patients, colleagues, or friends, Dr. Roberto Assagioli radiated joy, light, and positivity right up to the end of his life. He was passionate about making a difference in people's lives and believed we are all capable of finding that kind of unshakeable joy from deep within the self as we strive to reach our highest potential.

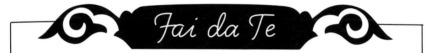

Fai da Te

CULTIVATE A SERENE MINDSET

One way to achieve serenity using the important tenets of psychosynthesis is to start with a small notebook. Divide the notebook (with tabs or bookmarks) into three sections.

Label the first section **Uplifting Words**. Fill as many pages as you need to using positive words that have meaning to you and that you would like to occupy your thoughts. Then write each word on its own index card, and place the cards throughout your home in the areas where you can't help but see them throughout your day.

Label the second section **Substitutions**. Here, you will keep a sort of log. Make two columns. Jot down the events of the present day that brought you down, made you feel sad, angry, anxious, or disgusted, in the column to the left. In the column to the right, record what you could do from here on in to substitute that negative thought or activity, replacing it with something that makes you happy or content.

Label the third section **Acting as If**. Each morning, set the tone of your day by envisioning yourself going through your day with joy and following your passion. Visualize the things you might do if you were living in the *bel paese*. Would you start your morning with a delicious cappuccino and fruit or chocolate-filled brioche? How about taking an after-dinner walk or *passeggiata* (weather permitting) and striking up some light conversation with the neighbors? Write out your best ideas for "acting as if" you are _____ (fill in with any mental or physical actions that will fill your heart with happiness and make your life sweeter).

18

La Moda Italiana

Italian Fashion

Italians know that clothes matter. How we dress affects how others see us, and more importantly, our appearance is a reflection of how we feel about ourselves. Confidence may be the most important Italian fashion accessory of all. It takes an ordinary outfit to a new level. Next on the scale of importance is good grooming. A good self-presentation is a sign of self-respect. On the streets of the *bel paese*, you will note the women walk tall, gracefully, and unhurried, almost as if inviting the admiration of observers. Men stride like peacocks, carefully dressed. Even when casual, their style is detailed with a hint of fine accessories.

You don't have to spend a lot of money to dress with an Italian flare. In addition to good posture (which is free), the key to looking expensive is to shop for quality clothing off-season, shop sales, or shop gently used designer pieces, but above all, choose items that fit well and flatter your individual body type. While it is important to purchase the best fabrics you can afford, less expensive pieces can be fitted by a tailor and made to look like you've spent a fortune.

Italian style is tastefully classic with a contemporary edge. A tailored blazer might be paired with a simple white T-shirt and jeans and accented with a beautiful neck scarf and large statement earrings. The women of ancient Rome used gold and pearl jewelry to illuminate their faces, and that tradition lives on. Gold chains, from the delicate to the bold, will never go out of style for both Italian men and women.

Beautiful lingerie is something Italian women wear for themselves, whether they have a partner who sees it or not. To get an idea of some extraordinary (albeit pricey) Italian undergarment designs, check out laperla.com. Italian women believe it is a sign of self-worth to purchase beautiful, soft, and comfortable feminine fabric and designs that fit close to the skin. The universal adage our mothers always told us holds true in Italy too: always make sure your undergarments are matching and in good condition, as you never know when you'll get into an accident!

Italy's fashion, like food, is serious business, going back to ancient Rome, when clothing conveyed status and influenced how one was treated. Roman women would spend hours on their hair, makeup, and choice of jewelry to accent their robes. Centuries later, Italian women (and men) still consider dressing style as an outward expression of *la bella figura* (putting one's best foot forward). *La moda* (fashion) is seen as an art form, the body being the canvas.

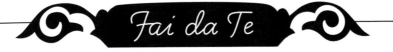

HOW TO DRESS LIKE AN ITALIAN

Since I was a little girl, the Italian women in my family taught me that it doesn't matter where we are going; we always feel better about ourselves when we dress up. Being well groomed and neatly dressed also reflects on the family as well as oneself. That is the principle behind *la bella figura*. The Italian women in my life taught me several fashion rules. Here they are:

Choose clothes that make you like how you look. When we treat our bodies with care and adorn them accordingly, we feel more confident.

Clothes can help you make a positive first impression. Whether you are going for a job interview or on a first date, an outfit you look and feel good in can be a helpful tool. In a large UK study, participants were rated more positively when dressed in more flattering clothing.

Shop quality items on sale. Made-in-Italy clothes draw admiration for their attention to the most delicate detail, the luxurious quality of their fabrics, and the innovative design that conveys classic with a slight edge without being trendy. Even in Italy, however, designer labels are respected though not absolutely necessary for a quality wardrobe.

Use good posture. Beyond the selection of clothing itself, standing up straight conveys confidence and personal power.

Jewelry should accent, not overpower. Gold hoops and button pearls are essential earring styles in every Italian jewelry box. Family heirlooms also provide a sense of belonging and connection to a woman's ancestry. Overdoing it with sparkle and jangle becomes more clownish than classy.

Wear a *foulard* (a neck scarf). Italian men and women are known for their love of scarves. Whether knotted loosely over the shoulder, double-looped at the base of the throat, or threaded chicly under the collar like a man's necktie, a scarf can bring an outfit to a whole new level, depending on the shape, fabric, and colors or prints you choose.

Keep your shoes clean and repaired. Accessories are those finishing touches that allow you to change the look of your outfit without having to keep buying new clothes. Footwear does the same. The Italian woman's shoe wardrobe essentials include basic black shoes or boots, delicate strappy stilettos for dressier events, and ballerina flats or loafers that can be worn with shorter (not mini) skirts and cigarette pants.

Carry an umbrella as a statement. A nice umbrella shows you take the time to care about your looks even when it rains! Since 1956, the brand Pasotti has been *the* name in luxury Italian umbrellas. If you want to see umbrella designs that take your breath away, take a look at their website, pasottiombrelli.com, and enjoy the magic. Whether vanilla cream with gold inner lining or plain black with gold studs around the edging and skull handle, Italian umbrellas make rainy days fashionable and elegant.

***Le borse italiane* (Italian handbags) can be beautiful and functional.** There are several leather schools and factories throughout Italy, particularly in Florence, but Pierotucci offers an online collection that is reasonably priced for rich, buttery leather (remember the feel of fabric is just as important as the style to the Italian way of thinking). Most women, especially if working outside the home, will own a laptop briefcase, a messenger-style bag, or a tote (replacing the traditional hard leather briefcase of yesteryear), such as the Toscanella red leather tote with lining. If you prefer not to purchase leather items (I don't), both faux leather and cloth handbags are great substitutes.

***Gli occhiali* (eyeglasses) are also important.** Eyeglasses were invented in Italy around 1285, and to this day, eyewear to Italians is considered as important as jewelry. Leonardo Del Vecchio started the Italian Luxottica eyewear company in the '60s, and it has become the largest eyewear company in the word. Its best-known brands include Ray-Ban and Persol. Luxottica also makes sunglass frames for Burberry, Versace, and Dolce & Gabbana, among other designers. And of course to all Italians, the sexy allure of a chic pair of sunglasses is a must!

Be bold, and wear *un cappello* (hat). In Italy, hat wearing is becoming a lost art, but for those who love to make a statement, hats still provide just the right touch of drama when one wants to get noticed. With over one hundred years of experience in hat design, the Florence-based Marzi family continues to be a formidable name in unique women's hats using materials such as straw, dried flowers, feathers, and various grasses as well as rich colors that turn a hat into a piece of artwork. Check out their beautiful designs here: marzi.com. As soon as you ascribe to the practice of wearing hats, you will undoubtedly command attention and admiration for your European fashion flair.

Fashion is fun and enjoyable. It allows you to be anyone you want to be. Don't be afraid to keep refining your image by updating your wardrobe.

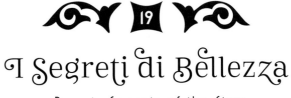

I Segreti di Bellezza

Beauty Secrets of the Stars

Italian bestselling author Dr. Piero Ferrucci believes that beauty has the power to change your life. Beauty is healing and uplifting, and we can find beauty everywhere if we look for it. Beauty can be discovered in nature, in music, in art, in the people we care about or admire, and in ourselves. The traits of kindness, generosity, empathy, gratitude, and appreciation might be thought of with respect to one's inner beauty. These qualities also translate to greater external beauty, which Italians believe is also important to attend to as part of their traditional *bella figura* philosophy of presenting oneself well. In Italy, tending to one's personal appearance is a sign of self-respect. It has also been linked to greater happiness, self-esteem, and psychological health.

Here are a few beauty tips for outer beauty that might be fun to try from the classic Italian stars of stage and screen:

Sophia Loren is the Italian film star most associated with timeless beauty. At the age of eighty-six, she returned to film to star in *The Life Ahead* and showed the world through her elegance and talent that beauty comes in all shapes and sizes and at every age. In her book *Women & Beauty*, Sophia wrote that a woman's beauty routine should not stop with the face. The skin on the hands, feet, elbows, and the rest of the body needs attention as well. The key is consistency, she wrote. The smoothing effects of using a pumice stone to rub away rough spots on your feet, for instance, can disappear if you are not consistent with your efforts. She also believes in setting up a home spa so you can pamper yourself. Some of the supplies to have on hand include bath oils (or salts), perfumed soap, a body brush, pumice stone, facial mask, body lotion, razor, and a transistor radio (translated to contemporary times, a favorite playlist on your smartphone). Begin by applying a facial mask and taking a nice leisurely bath using your fragrant soap. Rinse off in a cool shower; then follow with your favorite body lotion.

Claudia Cardinale, Italian actress and winner of beauty contests, was admired for both her talent and her nonchalant beauty. She had a captivating presence in Federico Fellini's 8½, and she never lost that grace and feminine beauty with the passage of time. In one interview, she shared her best antiaging beauty secret: "Stay active and never give up."

Gina Lollobrigida, referred to as the Italian Marilyn Monroe, was considered an international sex symbol of the 1950s and '60s. Until her death in 2023 at the age of ninety-five, she had an earthly glamour that came from taking care of herself and taking the time to plan out every detail of her wardrobe and accessories. In a 1950 interview, she emphasized the importance of natural-looking makeup, using olive oil to remove that makeup, and steaming her face with a hot towel afterward to clean the pores.

Virna Lisi, with an understated beauty compared to that of Sophia and Gina, starred alongside stars of both Hollywood (e.g., Jack Lemmon in *How to Murder Your Wife*) and the Italian cinema (e.g., Marcello Mastroianni in *Casanova 70*). Her classic '60s Italian beauty look included soft wavy hair, defined full eyebrows, and matte-black cat eyeliner, contrasted with a pale nude lip.

Monica Bellucci, star of the heartwarming film *Il Postino* (*The Postman*), is now in her fifties and is as breathtaking today as she was back when she starred in that film. She is a fan of the natural look, so when she chooses cosmetics, the colors are always earth-toned and muted. Fragrance is the finishing touch to her allure. Her favorite perfumes include Dolce & Gabbana's Sicily and Christian Dior's Hypnotic Poison.

Diego Dalla Palma, in his book *La bellezza interiore* (Inner Beauty), says it all in the title. Renowned makeup artist and cosmetic entrepreneur of made-in-Italy skin and hair products, Dalla Palma believes that real beauty has no age and is not exclusive to movie stars, because real beauty comes from the inside.

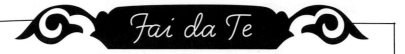

Fai da Te

HONORING YOUR PERSONAL BEAUTY

We are often so hard on ourselves that we become blind to our own personal beauty. To the Italian Catholic mindset, the fact that we are made in the image and likeness of God makes our beauty a given. Let's start here.

Make a list of your inner and outer qualities that are beautiful. If you can't think of any, then ask the people who love you most to give you a few descriptors. Beneath that list, jot down a few things you can do to take it a step further to enhance and highlight those beautiful inner and outer qualities.

Read the list every day so you will internalize it and stay motivated to continue to bring out those qualities. Italians don't believe in striving for perfection (as we all have human flaws), but they do believe in consistently working toward self-improvement and always putting their best foot forward. That is the Italian *bella figura*. Good self-care requires effort and consistency, but the reward is a boost in self-esteem, personal confidence, and greater life satisfaction.

La Donna Italiana

The Italian Woman

Italian women—in general—take loving care of their bodies, adore their children, and are devoted to their elderly family members. They live with passion, dress with tasteful flair, and in recent decades have made amazing inroads into areas that were once male-dominated in the workplace and in politics.

Traditionally when we think of important Italian historic figures, we think of Cicero, Dante, Vivaldi, Michelangelo, da Vinci, Galileo, Enrico Fermi, Marco Polo, Columbus, Silvio Berlusconi, Julius Caesar, and countless other men. But Italy is renowned for its culture, intellectualism, artisanry, and innovation because of the contributions of its women too. Feminism is thought to have actually originated during the Italian Renaissance with female writers beginning in the late fourteenth century exploring concepts of gender equality. Italy's brilliance lies in the accomplishments of too many women to name. Here are a few:

Dorotea Bucca (1360–1436) was chair of the department of medicine and philosophy at the University of Bologna in 1390. Italy has historically been more accepting of women in medicine, going all the way back to Trota of Salerno, a physician in the twelfth century and one of the first advocates of women's health.

Maria Montessori (1870–1952) was a physician and was also renowned in the field of education for her advocacy of the open classroom, where children were encouraged to move throughout the day while learning and given opportunities for hands-on manipulation of educational materials.

Artemisia Gentileschi (1593–1653) was an Italian baroque painter who apprenticed with her father, Orazio, and at the age of seventeen painted a scene from the Book of Daniel, *Susanna and the Elders*, that was so exquisitely and realistically done that she is still considered one of the most accomplished painters of all time.

Elena Cornaro Piscopia (1646–1684) was one of the first women in history to receive a university degree. She earned a PhD in mathematics at the University of Padova. A true genius, she was also an accomplished musician and played several instruments.

Grazia Deledda (1871–1936) won the Nobel Prize in Literature in 1926, honored in part for her inspiring and realistic depiction of life on her native island of Sardinia. A prolific and gifted writer, she wrote novels, short stories, plays, and poetry on themes of the human condition, such as moral dilemmas, passion, and temptation.

Rita Levi-Montalcini (1909–2012) was a Nobel laureate scientist and neurobiologist who codiscovered nerve growth factor. She overcame the oppressive forces of an authoritarian father who didn't believe in academic education for women as well as being a Jew in Fascist Italy. She eventually convinced her father to let her study medicine, as she could not let her gender hinder her from a professional career.

Isabella d'Este (1474–1539) is known as the First Lady of the Renaissance. From a young age, she could sing, dance, play musical instruments, and debate the finest politicians. Eventually she would become the mother of seven children as well as one of the most powerful, well-educated—not to mention well-dressed—political figures of her time. She was a great patron of the arts, commissioning both Titian and da Vinci to paint her portrait.

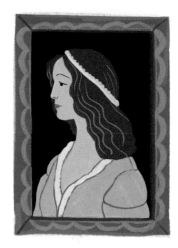

Not every accomplished woman goes down in the history books, but they do all share the passionate Italian approach to whatever they do. I learned the importance of taking pride in the details of one's work from my *zia* Rosaria, who wove baskets in the fields of Castelpagano; from cousin Concetta, who could needlepoint a portrait of Padre Pio as recognizable as a photograph; from my maternal grandmother, Geppina, who grew flowers that could rival those of anyone with a master's degree in horticulture; and from Angelina, my paternal grandmother, who ran a household, grew and canned her own food, raised five children, *and* became a small business owner with a mom-and-pop grocery store. These were the not-so-famous role models from whom I learned life's most important lessons. They were everyday Italian women who believed in themselves, made the best of any situation they found themselves in, and let hard work result in satisfaction and fulfilment. Researchers have found that we get the most lasting pleasure from the parts of life that require effort. Hard work gives us confidence, a sense of achievement, and a feeling of self-efficacy.

Fai da Te

IMMERSE YOURSELF IN THE DETAILS, WHATEVER YOU CHOOSE TO DO

To understand the soul of Italian women is to understand that passion, hard work, personal industry, and the courage to take risks all contribute to the cultural philosophy of a *lavoro ben fatto* (job well done).

Here are two ways that you can capture that spirit of the accomplished Italian woman:

1. Think of the activities or goals that you are passionate about. Write down your top three choices, along with a few ideas on the steps you must take to pursue these interests, and then work on them a bit each day. Perhaps you want to learn a new language, knit a sweater, write a novel, or start a charity.

2. Make each moment of your life count by devoting your full attention to it. Be fully present, no matter what job you do, no matter what tasks you have before you—even when you have to do the mundane, the boring, or the unpleasant. Honor your time by doing the best job you can, no matter how you feel about the task.

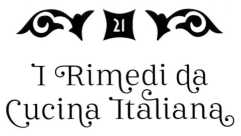

I Rimedi da Cucina Italiana

Italian Kitchen Remedies

One aspect of self-care involves visits to our physical and mental healthcare professionals as needed, but Italian grandmothers also believed there were many things we could do ourselves at home in the name of good self-care. They believed we had everything we needed for both beauty and good health right in our refrigerators or cupboards. A recent publication from the Italian publisher RIZA, called *I miracolosi remedi della nonna* (Grandmother's miraculous remedies), confirmed that our *nonne* knew what they were talking about! Highlighted are the following traditional Italian folk remedies as having the potential to improve both health and appearance:

Camomilla (chamomile): Once when in Calabria, Zia Bettina made my grandfather and me the most fragrant chamomile tea I've ever tasted. She had picked and dried the flowers herself, and as she steeped the little yellow and white blossoms, the fragrance was heavenly! A plate of homemade biscotti completed our *colazione* (breakfast). A change of pace from our usual morning cup of coffee, chamomile tea kept us calm and focused throughout the day. Italians have traditionally used chamomile tea to soothe digestive issues and to help with sleep. You can also squeeze out the cooled tea bags and place them over your closed eyes when you have a moment or two to recline. This will help make your eyes feel refreshed as well as decongest any puffiness around the eyelids.

Olio d'oliva (olive oil): Extra virgin olive oil, known as liquid gold in many Italian families, is believed to be a super antioxidant when consumed (for example as part of a salad dressing), but it can also be used as part of your self-care regimen. My Sicilian grandmother used olive oil on her skin as a moisturizer, and when mixed with a few sugar granules, it makes a wonderful natural scrub to exfoliate dead skin cells on any rough spots, such as elbows, knees, and feet. It is also great for dry hair. After washing your hair and before blow drying, you can take a few drops of oil, warm them up between your hands, and comb through the ends of your hair to keep them healthy and shiny.

Le fragole (strawberries): Italian grandmothers knew that strawberries are filled with natural vitamin C. Vitamin C has been said to boost collagen, fade hyperpigmentation, protect against sun damage and sunburn, and boost hydration. If you have a couple of ripe, organic strawberries, you can mash them and mix with a spoonful of plain Greek yogurt or honey, then apply to your face. Rinse off after ten minutes.

Il rosmarino (rosemary): It is believed that the herb rosemary is a great stress reducer. Either dried or fresh rosemary leaves, made into an infusion with hot water and drunk with a bit of honey two to three times a day during tense periods, is said to relax you. It may also strengthen fragile or thinning hair. Just make a mixture of mashed rosemary leaves with water or a bit of olive oil, and apply to your scalp, or use rosemary oil, diluted with a bit of olive oil if your scalp is sensitive. Leave on for ten to fifteen minutes, and then shampoo.

La salvia (sage): One of the few things that grow like wildfire in the suboptimal soil in my garden is salvia. These stately purple-flowered stalks are an old Italian remedy for inflamed skin, such as from an insect bite. Try rubbing the puncture with the salvia leaves. Or you can boil the flowers in water, and when the water cools down but is still warm, it makes a soothing foot or hand soak, a great way to unwind from a stressful day.

Le cipolle (onions): The onion has gotten a lot of positive press in recent times, mainly for its health benefits and ability to help keep illness at bay. The Italians of yesteryear used it as a common cold remedy. They would mash it, then take a small spoonful of the onion juice when they got the sniffles. Some also used it on the scalp to encourage hair growth.

L'aglio (garlic): Italians are often an unfair target of jest for their love of garlic (my father used to put a garlic necklace around our necks during flu season when we were young), but current research confirms that garlic is one of the healthiest vegetables one can eat. Italians believe it can also extend one's life. Some studies show that the properties in garlic can help lower blood pressure, aid digestion, improve blood circulation to the brain (which helps maintain sharpness), and even help temporarily soothe a toothache until you can get to a dentist. Of course, not everyone loves the strong flavor of garlic, so starting off with just a little bit is a good idea.

Il caffè (coffee): Beyond the benefits of drinking coffee in moderation, which we've discussed earlier, coffee grinds can also be used as a beauty remedy. Mixed with a bit of olive oil and rubbed onto areas of cellulite before a shower, it will make your skin feel smooth and silky.

Il limone (lemon): The lemons so big, juicy, and abundant along the Amalfi Coast can be squeezed and applied to your face or hands as a natural toner for nice, even skin and the reduction of the look of sun spots. It also gives skin a natural form of vitamin C. Wait a few seconds, and then rinse off with cold water. Do this daily.

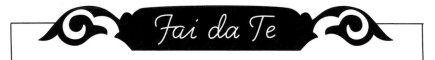

EXPERIMENT WITH FOLK REMEDIES

Have fun trying out one or more of these Italian folk remedies and see how they work for you. Also, ask the elders in your own family what natural kitchen ingredients they used for certain beauty or health issues. There is a reason that some of these age-old remedies never really get old at all!

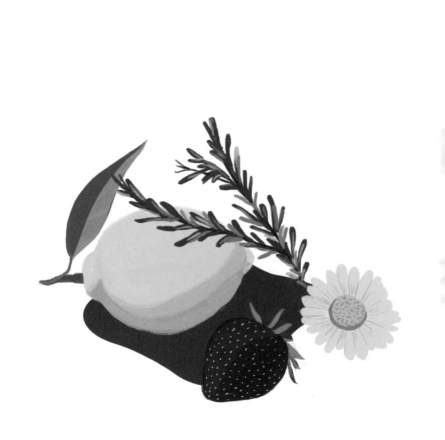

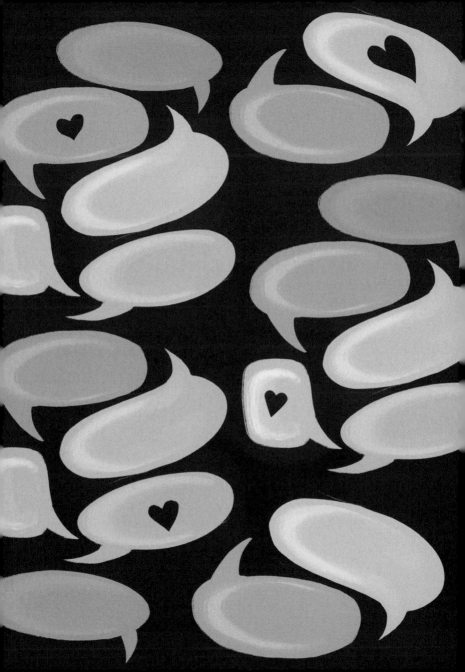

The Italian Celebration of Relationships

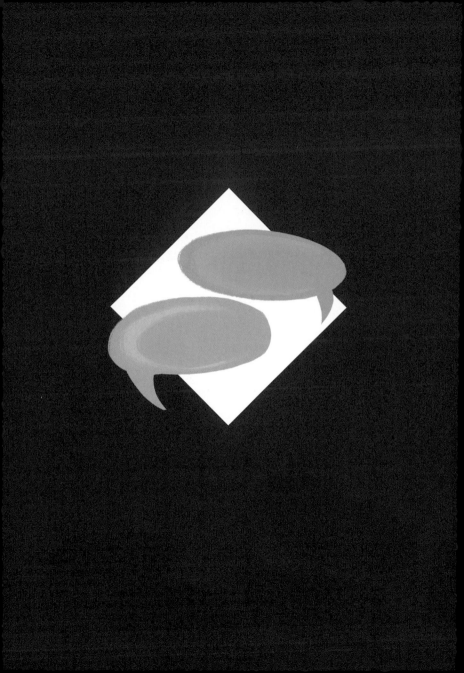

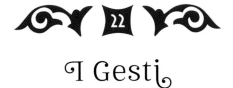

I Gesti

The Art and Value of Italian Hand Gestures

Whether born of the necessity to persuade crowds in ancient Rome or to be able to understand one another during times of foreign occupation—or even to compete for attention in a densely populated city—Italians have been using gestures to communicate for centuries.

One of the most brilliant communicators in world history was Marcus Tullius Cicero (106 BC–43 BC). A lawyer, philosopher, statesman, literary genius, and unquestionably one of the most eloquent orators of the Roman Republic, Cicero was sharp, knowledgeable, and verbally persuasive. He also believed that to deliver a speech of excellent quality, the message should be accompanied by "movement of the body," using "gestures, facial expression, and varying the inflection of the voice." Some likened this great orator to a theatrical performer—only even more captivating.

Research shows that gestures and verbal speech are dynamically intertwined. In ancient times, orators who received Roman rhetorical training were not only made to practice composition and writing style, but they also had to practice the delivery of the speech, a.k.a. the performance. Gesticulation was a crucial part of making that speech come to life. Moving the body from head to toe helped convey emotion and passion and captivate the attention of a crowd whom the speaker wished to move and persuade.

Marcus Fabius Quintilianus, born in Spain around 35 AD, was considered the first public professor of rhetoric (persuasive speech) and authored twelve volumes (*Institutio Oratoria*) on the education of an orator. He described in great detail every nuance that a public speaker should be concerned about. Examples included wearing the proper toga, memorizing one's written text, enunciating clearly, and practicing whole body delivery (including posture, hand and finger gestures) and learning which facial movements would help or damage the impact of the performance (i.e., one should never make movements with the nose while speaking).

A word about negative stereotyping: How many times have we seen Italians portrayed in the media with exaggerated, wild flailing of their arms? It's not that Italians *don't* talk with their hands; in fact, they produce *a lot* of nonverbal communication throughout the day—approximately 250 such daily gestures according to Italian communications expert Dr. Isabella Poggi. But what eludes the ridiculers is that Italian gesticulation is a sophisticated, culturally rich tradition, created to enhance communication, and is deeply rooted in the history of Italy and its people. Neapolitan-born archaeologist Andrea de Jorio (1769–1851) wrote an entire volume on the science of bodily expression and the connection between contemporary gestures observed on the streets of Naples and similar gestures uncovered in ancient frescoes during the excavations of Pompeii and Herculaneum. Italian body language is not a meaningless, random flailing of limbs and facial expressions but rather a complex and refined form of nonverbal communication for which Italians should be lauded rather than ridiculed.

Studies have found that even Italian children, from a very young age, display skillful gesturing likely from being immersed in such a gesture-rich culture. In fact, because of their tendency to include nonverbal communication skills when first learning to talk, Italian children were found to initially have smaller spoken vocabularies than American children of the same age. Those differences, however, quickly disappeared as the children got a bit older. Professor Poggi describes the lexicon of Italian gestures as comparable to the breadth and sophistication of sign language for the deaf. She believes gesturing first became popular in the busy southern Italian cities as a result of competition or as a way to stand out from the crowd.

Luigi Barzini, renowned Italian journalist and bestselling author, believed that Italians use gestures "more abundantly, efficiently, and imaginatively than any other people." They gesticulate when too distant to hear each other's words, when it is not polite to express something in words, or as a time-conserving technique, such as when a motorist doesn't want to slow down to shout insults to another motorist so instead might simply extend one hand in the direction of the other and fold all fingers except forefinger and little finger, making the shape of the infamous *mano cornuta*, or horned hand. Contrary to the negative media stereotype of exaggerated contortions of arms, hands, and fingers, Barzini describes the best Sicilian gestures as being "economical" and so subtle as to be almost imperceptible.

Sicilian actor, director, and author Luca Vullo tells the story of when he first moved to London and didn't speak a word of English. He used the "transcultural language" of Sicilian gestures to make himself understood. The response was overwhelmingly positive, and he now continues to spread the word about the richness and brilliance of the Italian gestural lexicon across the globe and in the fields of education and business. Thanks to the efforts of Dr. Vullo, the masterful art of Italian body language communication is helping people better understand each other, no matter what their background, culture, or mother tongue.

The moral of this story is that increasing our communication skills through the use of purposeful gesturing can help expand our social circles, and good interpersonal relationships are the strongest predictors of a happy life. Gestures and facial expressions can aid interpersonal understanding when you want to communicate with someone who speaks a language you don't know. They can help you communicate with someone with a hearing loss. They can help you hold an audience's attention when giving a speech or presentation. The use of appropriate hand gestures can be a great tool for building a bridge between you and others. Studies have found that gesturing is an integral part of communication. It conveys a link to speech and provides a depth of information that increases understanding among people, strengthens our social lives, and can help people with memory issues and communication disorders.

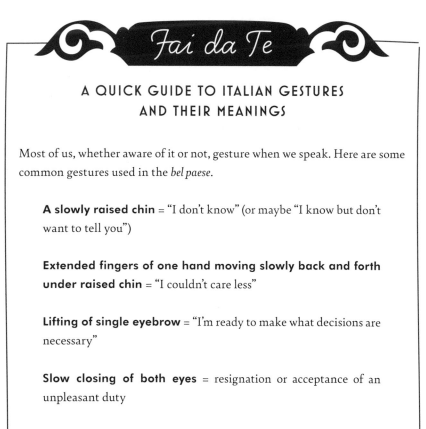

Fai da Te

A QUICK GUIDE TO ITALIAN GESTURES AND THEIR MEANINGS

Most of us, whether aware of it or not, gesture when we speak. Here are some common gestures used in the *bel paese*.

A slowly raised chin = "I don't know" (or maybe "I know but don't want to tell you")

Extended fingers of one hand moving slowly back and forth under raised chin = "I couldn't care less"

Lifting of single eyebrow = "I'm ready to make what decisions are necessary"

Slow closing of both eyes = resignation or acceptance of an unpleasant duty

***L'ombrello* (bent arm with fist, the other hand slapping the bicep of the bent arm)** = a rude way to say "go to hell" or something even more vulgar

L'occhio (the bottom eyelid slightly pulled down with your index finger) = "Watch out"

Index finger twisted into a cheek = "Delicious"

Palm facing up, fingers and thumb pinched together, rocking = "What do you want?" or "Who are you?"

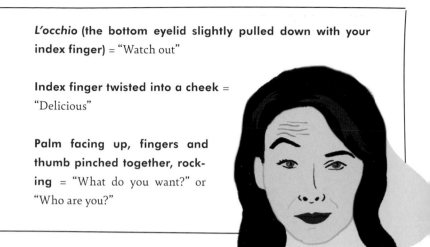

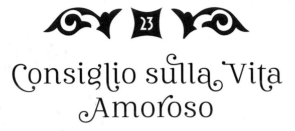

Consiglio sulla Vita Amoroso

Love Advice from the *Bel Paese*

If Cupid, the ancient Roman god of love, were ever to rename Italy, he would have to name it Amore. In fact, its capital city (Roma) spelled backward (Amor) supports this idea. Intimate relationships have been shown to reduce stress, lower blood pressure, and quench the human thirst for closeness to another human being. When we are attracted to another person, our brains produce oxytocin, the "happy hormone," which causes an increase in positive emotions. In other words, we feel better about ourselves and about the world around us. Love looms everywhere in the land of la dolce vita. Imagine cobblestone streets where centuries of people walked, emitting the electric charge of falling in love. Once the chemistry ignites, it may start with an informal *aperitivo* or an elegant dinner before the love poetry begins to flow as passionately as the waters of the Trevi Fountain. The lyrics would include the many ways afforded by the Italian language to communicate *ti amo* (I love you):

> *Ti voglio bene* (I love you, although this phrase is not quite as intense
> as *ti amo*)
> *Sono pazzo di te* (I'm crazy about you)

Non posso vivere senza di te (I can't live without you)
Sei il mio mondo intero (You are my whole world)
Sei la mia anima gemella (You are my soul mate)
Mi sono innamorato di te (I am in love with you)

Some of Italy's most historic cities are synonymous with love. We are all familiar with Verona, the setting for Shakespeare's *Romeo and Juliet*. Then of course there is Venice, a city that calls to mind images of Carnevale, nobility, gondolas—and love. And no surprise Venice is also the birthplace of Giacomo Casanova (1725–1798), serial seducer of women, whose love adventures are carefully documented in six thick volumes of autobiography.

Venice was also home to Zorzi (Giorgio) Baffo (1694–1768), who wrote erotic sonnets that were so licentious in Venetian dialect that I will refrain from reprinting them here. The plaque on the historic house where he lived says, "Here lived Giorgio Baffo, poet of love. He sang with maximum liberty and grandiose language."

Venetian society was also the setting for "honest courtesans," such as Veronica Franco (1546–1591), who became extremely wealthy by sharing their lovemaking skills with men of power and wealth. They were fabulously flamboyant dressers, adorned with beautiful jewelry and low necklines that offered just a peak at their sexy, silken breasts. Veronica, like many of her peers, was beautiful, educated, and classy. She even wrote poetry about the pleasures of making love:

> So sweet and delicious do I become,
> when I am in bed with a man
> who, I sense, loves and enjoys me,
> that the pleasure I bring excels all delight,
> so the knot of love, however tight
> it seemed before, is tied tighter still.

Valentine's Day is another gift of love and romance from Italy. San Valentino was a Roman priest believed to have lived in the third century. Legend holds that he married young lovers in secret, going against the law of Emperor Claudius II, who had outlawed marriage, decreeing that single men made better soldiers. Valentino was put to death for his actions around the middle of February, and thus the day of love was established to be February 14 and has been so ever since.

The concept of being *in* love was not always something that was considered in my grandmother's day, when marriages, especially in the south of Italy, were arranged. Practical partnerships of companionship and economic utility as well as the common goal of raising a thriving family were the greatest satisfaction one could desire. The simple pleasures of a close-knit *famiglia*, a warm bowl of *pasta e fagioli* after a hard day's work with a glass of *vino e pane fatti in casa*—these were the elements of true love to many Italians in an age gone by. Nothing wrong with a genuine, caring partnership no matter how a couple chooses to define it. Romantic love was only conceived of in more modern times. And Italy today is all about romance, as we can observe from the physical display of romantic expression across the streets and piazzas of the *bel paese*.

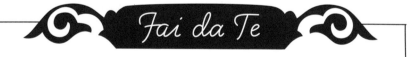

Fai da Te

LOVE ADVICE, ITALIAN STYLE

For some practical (and not so practical) Italian advice on love, here are a few perspectives from renowned figures from the *bel paese*:

OVID (43 BC–17 AD), the Roman poet, gave these pearls of advice:

On how to maintain one's appearance. Ovid believed we should try to look our very best. His ancient recipe for female beauty was to take two pounds of skinned Libyan barley and an equal measure of vetch (an herbal plant from the pea family). Moisten with ten eggs. Dry this mixture in "the blowing breezes," let the "she-ass" (female donkey) break it on rough millstone, then grind it with the first horns that fall from a nimble stag. Next, sift with a hollow sieve. Add twelve narcissus bulbs without their skins, and let a "strenuous hand" pound on pure marble. Add gum and Tuscan seed and nine times as much honey. Ovid promised that whoever shall treat her face with this "prescription" will shine "smoother than her own mirror." While you may not be off to the store in search of skinned Libyan barley, a more practical takeaway is to make sure the ingredients that you put on your skin do not include chemicals and preservatives that can harm it.

On where to find love. Ovid wrote, "Chance everywhere has power; ever let your hook be hanging; where you least believe it, there will be a fish in the stream." He also recommended women avoid those who profess "elegance and good looks" and who arrange their hair perfectly. It tells a woman that this kind of person may very well have had a thousand partners and is likely to wander.

On how to charm a woman. "Admire her arms as she dances, her voice as she sings, and find words of complaint that she has stopped. Oh, and take care not to show by your looks that you are feigning." (Note: Except that we women can usually tell a feigner!)

FRANCESCO ALBERONI (1929–) is an Italian journalist and sociology professor who described the phenomenon of *il colpo di fulmine* (love at first sight) as an imprinting that is often mistaken for true love. It may or may not be. Falling in love, he writes, is instead a process and goes beyond a singular initial fascination. Gradually, as love grows, there is a repeated experience of *un colpo di fulmine* as the couple continues to discover new and wonderful things about each other that they hadn't seen before. This is how true love grows.

LEO BUSCAGLIA (1924–1998) was a bestselling author and professor who created an entire course on love. While it is true that Italy as the home of Romeo and Juliet is the first country one thinks of when it comes to romantic love, love takes on a more encompassing definition in Buscaglia's view. He told us to love freely and, above all, to love ourselves. Most people, he felt, don't like themselves. When you think about it, the only thing you can give to anyone else is *what you are*. So make yourself the most wonderful and unique self you can be. You cannot be someone else, so develop yourself by learning something new every day. He also believed there is someone for everyone.

SILVANO ARIETI (1914–1981), an Italian psychiatrist who is still regarded as one of the world's foremost authorities on schizophrenia, presented readers with these rules when it comes to finding love:

- ✿ Overcome your personal fears about finding romantic love.

- ✿ Believe in self-worth and dignity, that you have a right to find love.

- ✿ Expose yourself to situations where you are likely to meet a partner.

- ✿ Don't look for the impossible or what is extremely difficult to find.

- ✿ Don't rush to accept or reject anyone. Love at first sight is a myth.

- ✿ Ask yourself why if you are rejected frequently.

- ✿ Don't misrepresent yourself.

❁ Don't expect success every time.

❁ Commit to finding love. Don't go about it half-heartedly but persevere.

And a bit of advice for those who have recently experienced a breakup and feel rejected:

FRANCESCO CAMPIONE (1949–), a physician, author, and clinical psychology professor at the University of Bologna, documented a few rules for healing from a broken heart:

❁ Distance yourself as much as possible and at least for a year from the person who doesn't love you, who no longer loves you, or who never loved you.

❁ Learn to be okay with loving yourself and appreciating the advantages of solitude.

❁ If someone doesn't love you, find someone else who does.

❁ Be happy with the love you feel in your heart. No one can take that away from you.

❁ If you feel anger or guilt over a love that is no more, give yourself time to get over these feelings, even if you need to get help to get over them.

Finally, consider the words of Roman emperor Marcus Aurelius: "When you arise in the morning, think of what a privilege it is to be alive— to breathe, to think, to enjoy, to **love**."

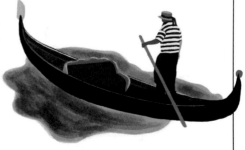

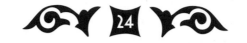

Fare Quattro Chiacchiere

The Italian Art of the Chitchat

If entire countries could be ranked on emotional intelligence (defined as the ability to understand human emotions and interact with warmth and empathy), certainly Italy would be at the top of the list, in part because of an unparalleled cultural skill in casual conversation. Italians see conversation as a colorful art form, punctuated by vocal dynamics, facial expressions, and appropriate hand gestures. *Fare due* or *quattro chiacchiere* (brief versus a longer chat) usually wraps up on a feel-good note, because Italians love to exchange pleasantries.

Yale psychologist Daniel Goleman, in his bestselling book *Emotional Intelligence*, described a New York City bus driver who was not all that different from what I observe every time I am with friends or family in Italy. It was a particularly hot summer day, and passengers were sweaty and grumpy as they boarded their bus with barely an expression on their face. The bus driver not only greeted each passenger with a welcoming smile and a cheerful line or two of personalized chitchat, but then he proceeded to turn what would have been a routine bus ride into a tour adventure for his passengers, pointing out the new restaurant that opened up here or the event that was going to be held there. By the time the passengers had to get off the bus, their whole demeanor had changed. They left with smiles on their faces that hadn't been there at the start of another humdrum day of routine.

The bus driver had what Goleman referred to as "emotional intelligence," something that traditional IQ tests can't measure. He had a personality that was upbeat, outgoing, and compassionate. He exuded happiness and cared to make other people feel happy too. This kind of social warmth is commonplace in Italy, and besides the food, when foreigners are asked what they found most memorable about their trip to the *bel paese*, they are quick to answer "the people."

Italians love people and love to talk to people, but that doesn't mean they don't express themselves honestly or their conversations are always light and superficial. If they do tell you something you don't particularly relish hearing (e.g., "that hairstyle is not the best for your face"), it is not coming from a mean place but rather a genuine attempt to be helpful. Take it as such. Albeit always ready to converse, Italians are not all that quick to trust strangers. One aspect of slow living—discussed earlier—is taking the time necessary to really get to know people in order to form deep and lasting bonds.

Florentine Italian, the standard language, became official in the fourteenth century with the work of Dante Alighieri, but over thirty-four distinct dialects and languages continue to thrive, especially within families, according to which region in Italy one lives. Then there are certain linguistic variations ascribed to the northern, central, and southern parts of Italy, with additional variations in vocabulary and pronunciation. Italy is a land of diversity when it comes to communication. That means talking *and* listening. Marcus Aurelius wrote, "Acquire the habit of attending carefully to what is being said by another, and of entering, so far as possible, into the mind of the speaker." In the classic book *How to Win Friends and Influence People*, author

Dale Carnegie wrote that listening and making someone feel they have your undivided attention is one of the most powerful tools of communication. Conversation is what keeps Italians connected with a fulfilling social life.

Fai da Te

SIMPLE WAYS TO MAINTAIN GOOD CONVERSATIONAL SKILLS

Italians are renowned for their people skills, the foundation of which is the art of conversation. Good communication is essential for acquiring and maintaining solid relationships along the course of our lives. Here are some ideas:

Try to see the glass as half-full. While some people look to find solidarity in complaining together, you can be the one to turn the conversation around by pointing out something positive you can all agree on.

Be well read. A person who reads is interesting. Read a wide variety of materials from celebrity gossip to medical newsletters and everything in between. Talk about a new novel or self-help book you read, and share the author's point of view. You will never have awkward silences if you stay informed.

Have an open mind to the ideas of others, and be curious. Ask questions. Everyone likes to offer their opinion. It makes them feel important to be asked their thoughts on a subject.

Be humble about your accomplishments; don't brag. Sharing your vulnerabilities endears others to you. It's called being real. For example, in Jerome Hines's book *Great Singers on Singing*, he describes interviewing the great tenor Placido Domingo. Hines complimented Domingo on his smooth transition into his high notes (a "cracking" voice is something many singers worry about and study for years to overcome). Instead of agreeing on how skilled he is, Domingo's response was one of innocent surprise. "Really?" he replied. Hines was charmed by how this amazing renowned talent was still so humbly focused on continued self-improvement, not self-aggrandizement.

Make the first effort to reach out to others. Talk to people who are waiting in line near you at the supermarket checkout or at the ticket window of the movie theater. It costs nothing to be pleasant, and you can very well make someone's day. Make eye contact (very important in Italian culture, as that is the way Italians gauge sincerity). Offer a smile and a cheerful word instead of walking past people without looking at them. Remember their name and they will remember you.

Stay neutral. Keep topics about politics, religion, or the gloom-and-doom news at bay, or you can easily get dragged into an unpleasant argument.

Show people you care about what they are saying. Look them in the eye. Nod in agreement. Rephrase what they have said so they feel heard. Share a similar experience.

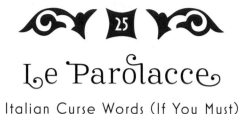

Le Parolacce

Italian Curse Words (If You Must)

Italians are passionate about family, food, love, and self-presentation. In fact, they are passionate, period! As such, every once in a while, the colorful Italian language will be peppered with the passion they have for interpersonal communication. According to communication experts, passionate people come across as genuine, authentic, and confident about the content of their message.

Once when I was dining with friends in a small town along the Amalfi Coast, the conversation got heated as an eighty-four-year-old woman began telling me how her ex-husband had been unfaithful. After a few profanities, she turned to assess my shocked expression and, with a look of satisfaction, confirmed, "*Beh, quando ci vuole, ci vuole*" (well, when it's necessary [to swear], it's necessary)!

Most everyone, whether Italian or not, knows a few Italian profanities. Many second- and third-generation Italian Americans will say they don't speak Italian except for the "bad" words, because when they were growing up, Italian was spoken in the home only when the adults didn't want the children to understand what was being said. Curse words are also often among the first words we mimic as children after hearing them from our parents.

While some Italians make an effort *not* to use *parolacce*, others admit to using such words regularly. Verbal vulgarities might be used in an argument, occasionally accompanied by a corresponding gesture. The emotions being expressed by *parolacce* don't always have to be angry, however. Curse words can also be uttered to express surprise or even a pleased reaction to something positive. *"Accidenti, che begl'occhi che hai!"* (Damn, what beautiful eyes you have!)

You might find it interesting to review some common Italian curse words that perhaps you have heard before. While this dimension of the vocabulary might bring color and emotion to this already rich Romance language, the following examples are for entertainment purposes only and not to be put to use. The point is not to advocate using curse words but rather to become aware of your own language and find ways to expand your vocabulary and put more cadence and energy into the way you express yourself. Passionate communication is not about yelling or cursing. It is about fully immersing yourself in the thoughts, ideas, and opinions you exchange with others. The truth is, only Italians themselves can use their *parolacce* without appearing foolish. When foreigners try to curse in Italian, it just doesn't have the same effect.

The Italian Curse-Word Primer

In case you happen to hear some of the following colorful expressions when you next visit the beautiful boot, you will now be able to interpret them.

Che culo!: typically means "What an ass!" (*culo* means "butt") but can also mean "How lucky!" depending on the intonation used and, of course, the situation.

Merda: "shit." One can say *"O merda,"* or *"pezzo di merda"* ("piece of shit").

Idiota/cretino: "idiot" or "jerk."

Bastardo/a: "bastard" in either male or female version.

Stronzo/a: "asshole" in either male or female version. Can be used in a joking way among good friends.

Che palle: literally "What balls," referring to the male testicles. However, when one uses this expression, they usually say it to mean something is boring.

Cazzo or **minchia (Sicilian form):** refers to the vulgar version of penis. This is one of the most common swear words used throughout Italy. One might say for example "*Quel libro di cazzo*" to mean "that crappy book," or "*Che cazzo vuoi*" to mean "What the hell do you want?"

Cavolo: literally means "cabbage," so it expresses a much tamer irreverence, such as "Damn!" or "*Che cavolo*" for "What the hell."

Figa: an impolite reference to a female part, so it is very vulgar. When someone says "*Che figa!*" it means "What a hot woman!"

Vaffanculo: we have all heard this expression, meaning "Go stuff it up your ass," or it is also used as a milder version of *fottiti* ("Go fuck yourself").

Coglione: a word meaning "big testicle." *Che coglione* would translate to "What a moron [or jerk]."

Rompipalle: "ball breaker." We need no example of how to use this in a sentence.

Figlio di troia: when used in a sentence, "son of a bitch."

Porca miseria: literally "pig [dirty] misery." When used in a sentence, this can be used to mean "Holy cow" or "Holy shit."

Now for the more **positive (non-curse) Italian expressions**, because it's always good to have a balance:

Bravissimo/a: "Very good."
Ce la fai: "You can do it."
Non mollare: "Don't give up."
Come stai bene: "You look great."
Auguri: "Congratulations."

Coraggio: "Have courage."

Forza: "Be strong."

Ti voglio bene: "I love you" (as would be said to a friend or family member).

Ti amo: "I love you" (as would be said to a lover).

Sei grande: "You're great."

Che bello: "How nice."

Sei bellissimo/a: "You're beautiful."

Che buono: "Delicious."

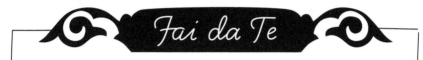

Fai da Te

LEARN ITALIAN

While *le parolacce* are fun and colorful, a foreigner using these words that are woven so naturally into the Italian vocabulary is not looked upon kindly. Better to use the more positive list, or take a beginner's course in the official Italian language. It is one of the most melodic and beautiful languages in the world! Italian is made up of dynamic intonations and open musical vowels. Try taking an adult language course or an online video course that teaches in a conversational way. One example is the podcast *News in Slow Italian*. But there are many others that even offer the possibility of supplementing your learning with a live language partner from Italy. A fun way to reinforce your learning is to watch Italian language movies on Netflix or subscribe to the Italian station RAI or Mediaset through your local cable company. You never know when you might get a chance to actually visit the *bel paese*, and if you do, you will see how thrilled Italians are to see you trying to learn their language.

ᴄᴇ 26 ᴇᴄ
ᴄᴇ Lezioni di Vita
Casanova's Lessons for a Passionate Life

Think what you will about him, and in many ways, he was certainly no role model, but Giacomo Casanova was a master in the art of seduction, which—negative connotations aside—can be an important tool in all areas of life. If wisdom springs from vastness of experience, deep reflection, and intellectual humility, we might come to appreciate the unexpected wellspring of insight from the oft-maligned personage of Giacomo Girolamo Casanova (1725–1798). Casanova was a man whose life was punctuated by euphoric highs and abysmal lows that most would have deemed insurmountable. Not for him. This prince of adventure always bounced right back in his quest to drink as much pleasure from the cup of life as possible, right up to the very last drop. Despite his strong Christian faith, he nevertheless abhorred—if not feared—the thought of dying without having concrete proof of a certain afterlife.

Casanova has gone down in history as an unabashed womanizer, doer of shady deals, gambler, swindler, and, at times, prisoner. Yet this same protagonist was also a university graduate, businessman, soldier, diplomat, and respected author and poet. He was sometimes welcomed by society and at other times banished from respectable circles (and sooner or later from most major cities in Europe as well!). This passionate Venetian lover was able to charm people (not only women) from every social stratum—from commoner to pope—with his *gioia di vivere* (never-ending resilience) and ability to easily

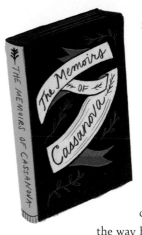

morph from one public persona into another. Ultimately, his was a lifelong quest to gain acceptance and respect while struggling to maintain balance between what Freud might call his instinctual drives versus his fragile capacity for self-control.

In his memoir *History of My Life*, written toward the end of his life, Casanova reflected candidly about his "errors," which resulted from being driven by his own curiosity. It is this very candor that makes us unable to pass judgment on the way he chose to live but instead leaves us rather grateful that he so freely shared what he learned. While unlike the typical religious or philosophical texts to which most people turn to be inspired, Casanova's self-analysis serves as a thought-provoking source of inspiration or at the very least provides an interesting look into the personal beliefs of a man the world was perhaps too quick to stereotype.

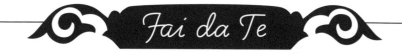

Fai da Te

THE LESSONS OF A LATIN LOVER OF LIFE

The following are some of Casanova's insights from his memoir. At the very least, they might serve as arguments to ponder. You might find that some points resonate with you. However, if you are in any way offended by his emphasis on God, it is perfectly permissible to skip this section, or simply read with an open, curious mindset.

We are free agents because God gave us the power of reason, and reason is a "particle of the Creator's own divinity." Destiny, on the other hand, Casanova believed, is a figment of the imagination. Belief in fate limits our power to be actors in our own lives.

Just because we are free does not mean we should do whatever we please. Casanova believed that we should use our reasoning power to make ourselves humble and just.

The wise person is not a slave to their passions but rather has the self-control to defer acting until calm. Casanova attributed his past errors to being a victim of his senses and acting more from feeling than reflection.

There is an immaterial God who answers prayers. This concept needs no explanation. Furthermore, there is plenty of research confirming the power of prayer.

Prayer kills despair. One should pray often, then trust that God will answer your prayers if you act accordingly. If you do so, you are never without hope.

Pray for grace; then believe you have received it, even if appearances seem to be the opposite. Casanova's inexhaustible optimism, as illustrated by this insight, was what both men and women found irresistibly charming about him.

Good comes from evil, and evil comes from good. Casanova believed that it is our job to straddle the ditch that divides the two sides of human nature. To do so takes not just strength but courage.

He believed that confidence without courage is useless. It takes courage to do the right thing.

One becomes a fool when in a fool's company. This serves as a reminder to choose the company we keep wisely. The people we surround ourselves with have a great influence on who we become.

Character shows up in the face. Casanova believed in a pseudoscience dating back to Aristotle called physiognomy. This is the belief that a person's personality, character, or temperament is revealed in their facial features or expressions. For example, a person with a high forehead would be considered intelligent. To the extent that it might be relevant today, one who frowns frequently might be seen as an unhappy person and vice versa. A good reason to smile often!

Hatred kills the unfortunate man who fosters it. Casanova admittedly found it easier to forget rather than forgive those who betrayed or mistreated him, but the bottom line was the same. He knew that anger, if left to fester, did more harm to the person holding on to it than to the transgressor.

Good food is important. While Casanova admitted to eating once a day to keep himself healthy, no one is recommending you do likewise, and in fact that is not the healthiest approach to good nutrition. Yet the importance of putting good-quality food into your body is a timeless bit of wisdom. Casanova also admitted to liking a nice dish of pasta, Neapolitan-style. If you ever get a chance to enjoy a delicious dish of pasta in Naples, Italy, I think you will agree!

Happy are they who know how to obtain pleasure without harming anyone. Quite endearing is the author's social consciousness. While admitting he was never a saint, he also deeply cared about the well-being of those he loved. This was evident in the way the women with whom he had affairs expressed a true affection for him.

"God demands only that we practice the virtues he has given us and has given us nothing which is not meant to make us happy." Casanova believed that some of our God-given virtues included self-esteem, desire for praise from others (also found in Maslow's hierarchy of needs), vigor (or practices that foster good health), courage, and moral freedom.

Life is the only treasure we possess, and those who do not love it do not deserve it. This too is self-explanatory, advising us of the importance of not taking life for granted.

Self-love is important. "I have always admitted," wrote Casanova, "that I was the chief cause of all the misfortunes which have befallen me. I have rejoiced in my ability to be my own pupil and in my duty to love my teacher."

To be human is to live a life of peaks and valleys as we strive toward continual self-betterment. Casanova, in allowing us to become observers in the open theater of his life, reminds us we are not alone in our struggle—as St. Augustine knew all too well—to avoid temptation and stay (as best we can) on the path of virtue.

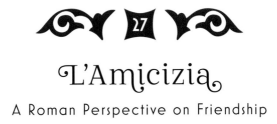

L'Amicizia

A Roman Perspective on Friendship

Most Italians when asked what they like to do during their leisure time, will tell you they like to spend it with friends. And because many remain in their hometown for life (often in the same house in which they were raised), they enjoy lifelong friendships going back to their childhood school days. There is a very common and classic Italian saying: "*Chi trova un amico trova un tesoro*" (When you find a friend, you have found a treasure). My grandfather would add "*I veri amici si contano sulle dita di una mano*" (your **true** friends can be counted on the fingers of one hand). If family is the sturdy outer shell of a house, friends are the furniture, appliances, and decorations. We know from the research that having friends can extend the length and quality of our life. Moreover, a healthy social life can protect against depression and loneliness.

Friendships sometimes end, however, for a number of reasons. People move away, change jobs, die, or just stop talking to each other. Apart from unavoidable circumstances, friendships, like gardens, require effort to maintain them. Deep friendships need time, touch, and eye contact. Virtual relationships are fine, but Italians usually prefer to connect in person. Someone I know recently remarked that she just returned from her first vacation in Italy. When I asked what she liked most about her trip, she stated two things: the slower pace of life and the easy way people interacted. Said my friend, "It seemed like a culture where people don't spend all day and night locked up in

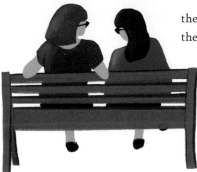

their rooms on social media, but instead, they are out everywhere chitchatting, walking arm in arm, laughing, and just sharing life. Even the waitstaff at restaurants are interested in getting to know a little bit about you. People look you in the eye when they pass you on the street or in the square. They don't just keep their head down and keep going."

Making and keeping friends is a lifelong process, and who better than the Roman philosophers to give us timeless friendship guidelines that inspire us even today. Here are a few of their perspectives.

Marcus Tullius Cicero (106 BC–43 BC) was a lawyer, philosopher, statesman, and defender of the Roman Republic. He was also an eloquent writer who wrote timeless and moving treatises on topics that are vital to our well-being. One of these was a letter he wrote to his best friend, Atticus, revealing his thoughts on "How to Be a Friend." It is still considered one of the best works on this subject of all time.

Cicero acknowledged that we form friendships for all kinds of reasons. Some relationships are utilitarian, meaning they are mutually beneficial in some way. There is also a *deeper* type of friendship, where neither party is seeking to profit in any way from the other. Cicero emphasized the importance of appreciating the people in our lives, not for what they could give us but simply because they are kindred souls. He wanted us to keep a few specific points in mind with respect to friendships:

- ✿ Friendships come in all shapes and sizes and are formed for a myriad of reasons. Some might be neighbors, coworkers, etc., but those few deep friendships (the ones we can count on the fingers of one hand) can be life changing for both parties. They are rare because they require effort in the form of time and attention to maintain them.

❀ Keep in mind that good people can be true friends. Cicero wrote abundantly on the importance of morals. Friendship, he believed, requires trust and goodness. He also advised us to take time in forming friendships so we can get to know each other on a deeper level. Otherwise, it may end in a painful break of the relationship when we realize that person is not the person they appeared to be.

❀ Among the stateman's wise advice, he wrote that cultivating friendships, although they may change over time, is nevertheless worth the time and effort it takes, as life without friends is not worth living.

Cicero was not the only Roman philosopher who deemed friendship an important topic to address; the Stoic Seneca the Younger (50 AD–65 AD) also documented, in epistolary form, his insights on the subject. In *Letters from a Stoic*, he pointed out that with a true friend, you can feel free to talk about anything. Once a friendship is established, it requires the trust of both parties, but when the friendship is still initially being formed, keen judgment is required. Some people get that sequence wrong, which leads to ending up with a "false friend." We might trust too easily, then judge the person to discover they are not worthy of our trust. Seneca believed that while it is natural to want friends, we must not forget that we alone are still the sole creators of our own happiness. He uses the metaphor of losing a limb and learning to adapt and be happy without that limb, even though we would have preferred not to have lost it in the first place. Similarly, sometimes "fair-weather friends" will desert us, and in the end, we should accept that with equanimity, because it was probably a friendship of utility. Once the other party got what they wanted, nothing can stop them from leaving, but we never have to lack friends if we make the effort to keep making new ones. One important step toward making real friends is to work on *ourselves* so that we are truly capable of giving and receiving the kind of love exchanged in deep friendships.

Fai da Te

TAKE A FRIENDSHIP INVENTORY

One of Italy's most famous singers, Gianni Morandi, had a hit song called "*Il Mio Amico*" in 2003. The lyrics exquisitely express how having this close friend changed his life, taught him how to appreciate the beauty in life, and cheered him up when he felt down, without expecting anything in return. How many *true* friendships do you have in your life? Can you count them on the fingers of one hand, like my grandfather would say? Here is how to take stock of your friendship circle and assess what needs to be done to have a happy long life, powered by friends who care about you.

On a piece of paper, list your very truest friends and all the qualities you love about them. If the list is too short or if you find you don't have one or two close friends, make plans to go out to places and events where you will likely meet the kind of people who share your interests. Start conversations by exchanging pleasantries, and decide whether to initiate further contact, perhaps grab a coffee, *aperitivo*, or gelato together. The Roman philosophers taught us that friendships are important, they take time to develop, but they are never a *waste* of time. Although it is true that we are responsible for our own happiness, life is much more enjoyable when we have friends to spend our leisure time with, just as they choose to do in the land of la dolce vita.

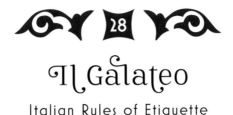

Il Galateo

Italian Rules of Etiquette

How many times have you witnessed or been the recipient of a door that was not held open for you by the person ahead? What about offering to let another car go first when at an intersection and you get neither a nod nor a wave of thanks? Perhaps you have been just about to take your place in the supermarket line when someone pushes in front of you without asking or excusing themselves. Rudeness and incivility seem to be so diffuse they are becoming the norm. Hardly anyone is surprised, and yet you rarely hear teachers, public speakers, or even preachers talk directly about the importance of manners and civility. Good manners include being kind, respectful, polite, and thoughtful toward your neighbor or toward a stranger you pass on the street.

Among my treasured collection of Italian books is *Galateo*, written by Giovanni della Casa in 1558. It is one of the first guidelines on social behavior and manners. Psychologists have found that manners play an important role in getting along with each other. Manners are about being kind, courteous, and compassionate, all of which wins the esteem of others, lowers stress, and improves social relationships. Della Casa's social etiquette guidelines cover all aspects of proper behavior—from how to eat to how to dress. He believed all tasks should be done well and with gracefulness. When one talks, they should be well informed before speaking. Posture is important, and one's walking pace should be neither too fast nor too slow.

A more contemporary proponent of the importance of good manners is Pier Massimo Forni (1951–2018), who was an Italian literature professor at Johns Hopkins. He authored the bestselling book *Choosing Civility: The 25 Rules of Considerate Conduct*, which essentially reflected an argument against rudeness. Dr. Forni believed that civility, which involves courtesy, kindness, and good manners, is a code of decency that should not be an abstract philosophical concept but rather a set of rules that should be applied to everyday life. Civility is not only a social responsibility, but it also enhances the quality of life. Life is difficult enough. Acting with kindness, the author believed, lessens life's burden for others. Also, the way we treat others is a measure of our own success. If you want to improve your relationships, it might be useful to brush up on a few basic Italian rules of etiquette.

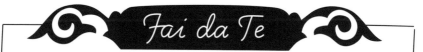

Fai da Te

AN ETIQUETTE REFRESHER

Kindness and civility go a long way in creating happiness for others, as well as for oneself. The Italian respect for life is displayed by acting with dignity and grace. Here are some examples:

- ❉ Dress neatly and appropriately.

- ❉ Do not eat until your host/hostess is seated and invites you to eat by saying something like *buon appetito*.

- ❉ Hold doors open for your elderly loved ones.

- ❉ Do not put elbows on the table while eating, nor wear a hat.

✿ Do not leave your mouth uncovered when sneezing or coughing.

✿ Make pleasant conversation.

✿ Always have something to eat on hand to offer unexpected guests.

✿ Look people in the eye when you raise a glass to make a toast (and never with an empty glass).

✿ If you are a dinner guest, bring wine, chocolate, or flowers—but not chrysanthemums, which in Italy are considered funeral flowers.

✿ Respect your elders by giving up your seat on the bus or standing up when they enter a room, and if you know them well, you may address them as *zia* or *zio*.

✿ Do not take off your shoes when you enter someone's home (unless you are asked to do so), but do wipe your feet thoroughly on the mat at the entrance.

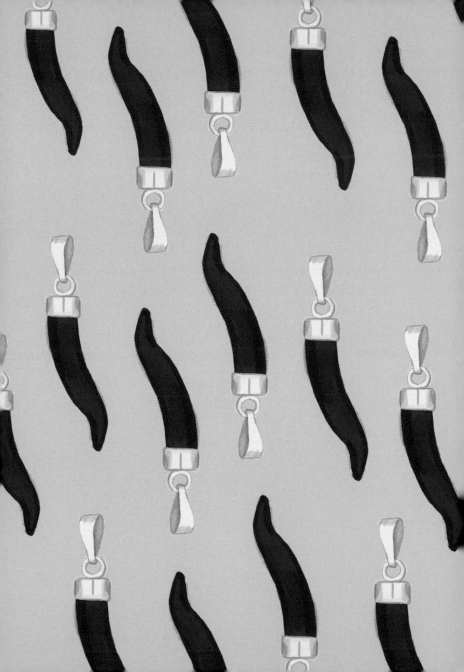

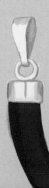

The Italian
Celebration
of Beliefs

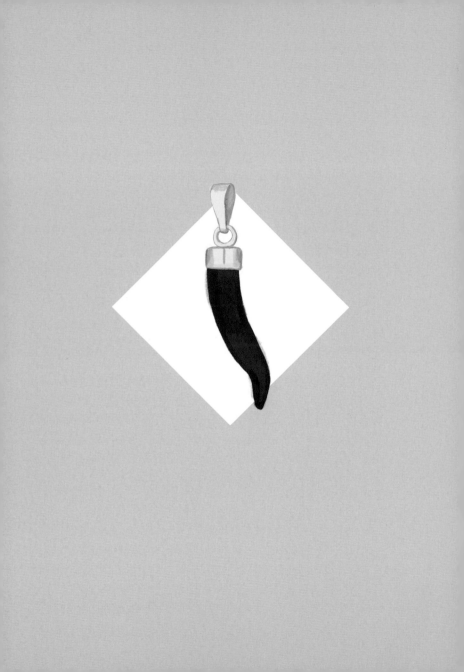

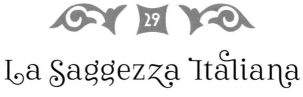

La Saggezza Italiana

Italian Wisdom for Living

Italians have inherited a centuries-old template on how to live well. The characteristic sweet life may be in their ancestral DNA, but it is not exclusive to those blessed enough to live in the *bel paese*. I wrote this book to prove that *all* of us—no matter our geographical, ethnic, racial, religious, or gender specifics—can make our lives more meaningful, more satisfying, and more dolce. One way to realize this goal is to consider the wisdom of the ancient Roman philosophers and other celebrated figures who continue to inspire the world centuries later with their contributions. Here are some life lessons that inspire me in my daily life and that might inspire you too.

General Wisdom

Leonardo da Vinci, by example of his insatiable curiosity, teaches us to learn everything we can as a road to personal development. He had to experience firsthand how water flowed and how birds flew. He spent hours sharpening his observational skills, which today has become a main methodology for conducting research.

Dante Alighieri, in his *Divina Commedia*, invites us to follow the protagonist from the depths to the heights of human experience. This magnificent work has given countless readers the courage to know they can rise from their own personal Inferno, up through the transitional state of Purgatory, and eventually arrive in a place of Paradiso. Several contemporary self-help books have been based on Dante's *Divine Comedy*.

Marcus Aurelius, often called the "good emperor," wrote of his gratitude for the people who influenced his life—past and present. He acknowledges each lesson he learned from family members, friends, teachers, and acquaintances. We have learned many lessons—good and bad—from the characters who have come in and out of our lives. From their examples, we learn to become who we are, what we aspire to be, and what we refuse to become at all costs.

Seneca, the Stoic Roman philosopher, taught us that a serene life is a result of accepting reality with fortitude and self-control. Meditation is based on the principle of being in the present moment and accepting what is instead of ruminating over the past or worrying about the future.

Giacomo Casanova, for whatever his flaws in the realm of romance, certainly serves as an example of the power of charisma. Through his suave self-confidence, women by the droves wanted to be with him, and men wanted to be him. The secret of his charisma was to have a broad enough knowledge base to be an interesting conversationalist and above all to make each person feel like *they* were the most interesting person in the world.

Marcus Tullius Cicero comforts our fears about growing old. "Old age," he wrote, "can be a wonderful part of life." When an older person is unhappy, the number of years that person has lived is not the culprit. A lack of internal resources is more likely to be the cause.

Ovid, the Roman poet, laid out a template for what Italians do best—*amare*, love. In *The Art of Love*, he advises a man to make it a priority to compliment the woman he loves: "be sure she thinks you are spellbound by her beauty." What woman—or man for that matter—doesn't want to be made to feel they are special in the eyes of the person they love?

Finally, every Italian I know associates **St. Francis of Assisi** with the important trait of altruism and with the virtue of giving.

Lifestyle Wisdom

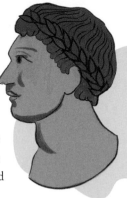

The Romans gave us the concept of making **meal-time** not just a necessary refueling but rather an important event to be enjoyed in company whenever possible. Extra-special dishes were brought out for guests. Three or more courses were offered in dining halls (triclinium) furnished with comfortable couches, artwork on the ceilings and walls to provide visual beauty, and the food and drink would be served in exquisite goblets and bowls.

Italians today still prefer to break bread in company. In my grandmother's house, we never knew who would show up for the midday meal. Anyone in the family who happened to pay her a visit around mealtime had a place set for them. Likewise, any neighbor who smelled the delicious aromas when the windows were open would be invited to join. Mealtime was much more than food, although good food was the cornerstone. It was also about love and caring and sharing what you had.

The priority placed on **self-care** dates back to ancient Roman society. The ritual of the Roman baths, for example, served as a vehicle to rejuvenate the body. One would undress in the apodyterium, or dressing room, where shelves would store one's clothing. Next off to the palaestra, or open-air exercise garden, where one could play ball, lift weights, or throw a discus. From there, the body would be oiled before taking a cold plunge in the frigidarium, then directly to the tepidarium, which was a pleasantly toasty room, heated by an underfloor heating system. Next came a room with a hot plunge bath, and finally any remaining oil was scraped off the skin. No cutting corners here! Most of us rarely spend more than a few minutes a day on caring for our bodies.

Recreation played an important part in ancient Roman life, reminding us how important it is to make time for carefree fun. Games such as chess, ball toss, and checkers as well as sports and entertainment like chariot races were popular.

Humans have valued the **arts** since the beginning of time. It is said that prehistoric humans drew, painted, and carved for aesthetic reasons. Art seems to be a necessity for the soul. **Literature**, from poets like Ovid, Virgil, and Horace, was widely appreciated, as was **music**, which played a part in every centuries-old event, reminding us how very human and dolce it is to nurture our artistic sensibilities.

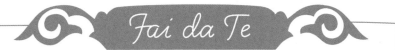

Fai da Te

SEVEN WISE WAYS OF LEONARDO DA VINCI

Take notes on your life. Leonardo not only left us the gift of insight into his genius through his notebooks, but he developed his own intellectual, scientific, and artistic skills by writing down everything that came to mind. He started in his thirties, but unfortunately most of what he wrote has disappeared. What remains shows architectural drawings, practical military designs, memos, sketches, personal notes, and a developing philosophy of the world through simple observation, the basis of our scientific method today.

Be curious about everything you observe. In modern terms, this is called mindfulness. Take in the wonder of the sights, sounds, and smells of your world. Pay attention to detail, and you will notice how time no longer has the power to fly by without your knowing where it went.

Diversify your interests. Leonardo's notebooks provide evidence of his interests in drawing, painting, sculpture, anatomy, optics, engineering, astronomy, and more. In our short lifetimes, most of us tend to narrow our fields of learning.

Learn reality from nature. Leonardo, unlike many of his illustrious contemporaries, did not have the luxury of a formal education. No one can refute his genius, however. From the time he began to explore the countryside as a little boy, his love of nature taught him how to look scientifically and objectively at the world around him. We spend the majority of our time indoors. We go from home to work, back to home or to indoor meetings and events. Make it a point to step out more into the outdoors. Go barefoot if you can, and ground yourself in the energy of the earth. Stop whatever you are doing to enjoy a rainbow. Notice how the insects, birds, and squirrels go about busily playing, foraging for food, and taking care of matters in their daily life.

Develop skills that will help both others and yourself. When Leonardo wrote a letter to the ruler of Milan seeking employment, he promoted his skills in the order in which they would be most useful in that zeitgeist, starting with his military engineering capabilities. Many college students are misguided in taking courses that upon graduation will leave them with mountains of debt and no employable skills that would help pay back that debt. Get some guidance from a trusted source if you are not clear on what direction you want to take your studies or career.

Think for yourself. It was no secret that Leonardo was not able to read Latin, and therefore despite his efforts to teach himself the language that all men of letters and science used, his struggle was real. He reasoned that experience was even more important in bringing about wisdom.

Emulate the masters. We might call it apprenticeship, a process that has been all but lost over the centuries. Leonardo advised young painters to first learn perspective, then proportions, then copy from a good master.

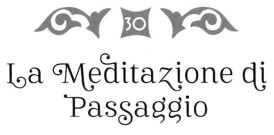

La Meditazione di Passaggio

The Power of Passage Meditation

Italy is the land of Dante, the literary genius of the late medieval period whose greatest work, *The Divine Comedy*, is still read and analyzed all over the world today. It is also the birthplace of Renaissance poet Francesco Petrarca (Petrarch), who, in addition to penning his treasured love sonnets, wrote one of the first and most popular self-help books of all time, *De remediis utriusque fortunae* (Remedies for fortunes), where he introduced the idea that our thoughts and actions can either make us happy or miserable. Other literary heavyweights of the *bel paese* include Giovanni Boccaccio (*The Decameron*), Niccolò Machiavelli (*The Prince*), Alessandro Manzoni (*The Betrothed*), and countless contemporary writers, leaving Italy with no shortage of inspirational reading material.

The benefit of reading not only for learning or entertainment but also for inspiration is not lost on Italians. Certain passages have the power to calm, encourage, motivate, and inspire. They can also serve as an alternate way of meditating.

Experts often recommend meditation to reduce stress and increase mental and physical well-being. I once taught several stress-reducing meditation techniques to cardiac patients who were participating in a large research study at Yale University. They were able to then use meditation and relaxation techniques to keep calm when faced with nerve-racking challenges or when they had to make big decisions.

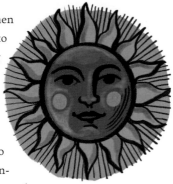

While it has been established that meditation is good for us, we don't always realize that it can take various forms that go beyond sitting cross-legged and chanting mantras or trying to empty the mind for hours on end. The beneficial effects of meditation can be acquired through visualization, prayer, or even a mindful nature walk. Lesser known is the powerful effect of meditating on an inspirational reading passage. The passage you choose to reflect on is anything that resonates with your current situation or state of mind. You might find serenity in reading poems or the writings of your favorite philosopher. Even a good self-help book can provide calming inspiration.

Researchers believe we become what we give our attention to. Albert Bandura, renowned for his theory on social modeling, knew there was more to learning than just trial and error from direct experience. The settings we live our lives in provide us with limited experiences. We travel in narrow circles and within the confines of daily routines. Thus, much of our learning about how to be in the world comes vicariously—including from the materials we choose to read. Passage meditation helps us live more deeply and get a better sense of who we are.

Once on a train back to Napoli to visit family, I turned to a book written by one of Italy's most treasured authors, in the area of psychospirituality. The book was *Come attraversare la sofferenza e uscirne più forti* (How to overcome suffering and come out of it stronger) by psychoanalyst and professor Dr. Valerio Albisetti. As I thumbed through the pages, one passage stood out, and unbeknownst to me, it would continue to inspire me whenever I face a challenge. The passage (and I paraphrase) went in part like this:

Quando soffri...
Quando ti senti dolore...
Entra nel profondo del tuo CUORE.
Lì vi troverai l'energia, la Luce per poter continuare.

When you suffer...
When you feel sorrow...
Enter into the depths of your HEART.
There you will find the energy, the Light to be able to
continue.

This is one of my favorite passages to this day, and I reflect on it often.
It never fails to bring me inner strength and tranquility.

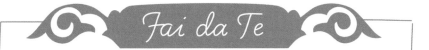

Fai da Te

EXPERIMENT WITH PASSAGE MEDITATION

If we do indeed become what we give our attention to, now is the perfect time
to bookmark a few readings to reflect upon with regularity.

Passage meditation, as it is called, can provide a powerful tool for inner peace
and spiritual well-being, whether you ascribe to a particular religion or not.
Start with a passage that has personal meaning for you, one that mirrors the
values with which you identify. Read the passage several times, or memorize
it; then sit in a comfortable position, close your eyes, and contemplate the
meaning of the words in that passage. Don't get distracted by word associations. Bring your full attention back to the passage if your mind wanders.

La Creatività

The Gift of Creative Genius

One of the biggest obstacles to creativity is the inability to break out of rigid routines. Habitual living keeps us from thinking outside the box and kills curiosity. Yet the world *needs* creative thinkers. Creative thinkers are who got humans to fly to the moon, cure diseases, compose artistic masterpieces, and come up with innovative ways of doing things, as in the layering of light technique that da Vinci used in painting the *Mona Lisa*.

The ancient Greeks and Romans believed that creativity came from the gods, and if that is the case, then Italy must have a direct heavenly line. Think of the musical genius of Vivaldi and Verdi; the fashion innovations of Prada, Versace, Armani, and Ferragamo; the invention of laws, pizza, pasta, the Vespa, the Ferrari, and the Maserati; the art of Michelangelo; the designs of da Vinci; the innovations of Montessori, Galileo, and Dante. The list goes on and includes the artisanry of Murano glass blowers, the cameo carvers from Torre del Greco, and the porcelain Capodimonte artisans from the Naples region.

Italians were among the

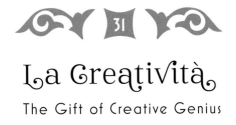

first to give us the idea of banks (Giovanni di Bicci de' Medici founded the Medici Bank in 1397), the first newspapers (in sixteenth-century Venice), the piano (invented by Bartolomeo Cristofori in 1700), the radio (Guglielmo Marconi), the calendar of Julius Caesar (slightly modified by Pope Gregory XIII), and the love sonnets of Ovid. Add to that the parachute, the jacuzzi, the battery, and much more.

We all have the potential to develop our inner creative genius, and if we fail to nurture it, we deprive ourselves and the world of our potential contributions big and small. Creativity often blossoms when you pursue activities you really love doing. Do you like to write songs? Bake cookies? Play an instrument? Design fashions? Compete in sports? Try your hand at new inventions? Whatever makes your soul come alive, you must first learn all you can about it. Read, take classes, or find experts in the field who will mentor you. Read biographies of people you would like to emulate, and follow their blueprint for success.

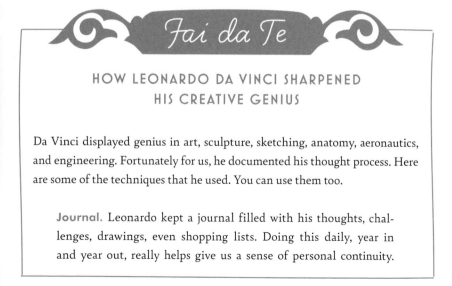

Fai da Te

HOW LEONARDO DA VINCI SHARPENED HIS CREATIVE GENIUS

Da Vinci displayed genius in art, sculpture, sketching, anatomy, aeronautics, and engineering. Fortunately for us, he documented his thought process. Here are some of the techniques that he used. You can use them too.

Journal. Leonardo kept a journal filled with his thoughts, challenges, drawings, even shopping lists. Doing this daily, year in and year out, really helps give us a sense of personal continuity.

Leonardo recorded thousands and thousands of pages, which contemporary research confirms can help us keep track of challenges and successes and increase motivation and focus. He developed his own intellectual, scientific, and artistic skills by writing down everything that came to mind.

Creative time should be spent alone. Leonardo warned that when you are alone, you are your own master, but when you are in company, your attention is divided. You are much more likely to be able to concentrate and come up with new ideas when you have some undisturbed time.

Trust your own experience. Da Vinci admitted that while he had no formal education, he found it more worthy to rely on his own efforts and experience rather than solely on the works of others.

Persist. Everyone has failures and problems that seem insurmountable when pursuing their dreams. Pick yourself up and keep going. Success comes to those who get up as many times as they get knocked down. "Obstacles cannot crush me," wrote Leonardo. "Every obstacle yields to stern resolve."

Learn and keep learning. Leonardo believed we can neither love nor hate what we don't first know about. All knowledge is useful, and a creative mind always seeks to know more.

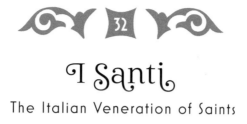

I Santi

The Italian Veneration of Saints

Not all Italians believe in saints to the same degree, but whether they're seen from a religious or a secular perspective, most won't deny that the lives of saints are templates for exemplary lives of virtue, love, and holiness. They are to be emulated. We speak to them to intercede on our behalf when we need their help, want to make a request, or just need a miracle.

Sore throat? Time to invoke St. Blaise. Lost car keys? St. Anthony to the rescue. Pet dog sick? St. Francis, hear our prayer. In the Italian culture, specifically among Catholics, various saints are also believed to protect against snake bites, spousal abuse, stiff joints, ulcers, and whooping cough. Some saints protect whole towns like Agrigento, Amalfi, and Rome. Professions and trades are also watched over by saints. St. Joseph (San Giuseppe), earthly father of Jesus, was a carpenter and thus the patron saint of workers. His feast day, March 19, is celebrated in Italy as Father's Day. The Tavola di San Giuseppe (St. Joseph's Table) is a custom believed to have originated during the Middle Ages in Sicily, following a famine caused by a severe drought. The people prayed to St. Joseph, and it rained. In gratitude, every year on March 19, the people of Sicily prepare outdoor tables of breads, pastries, and pastas to feed the less fortunate of the village. Offerings might include cream puffs (*zeppole*) as well as pasta with chickpeas and spinach and also special *pane di San Giuseppe* (St. Joseph's bread), artistically shaped in the form of a cross, chalice, heart, or ladder.

Foreigners seem fascinated with Italy's veneration of the saints, but to Italians, these half-human, half-divine beings are a normal part of daily life, offering spiritual inspiration and moral support and making one's faith more tangible. Every saint has led a life of courage, suffering, and divine human strength. Having once been human, they have had earthly hurdles to overcome and passions to pursue. In reading their biographies, we discover similarities to ourselves. From their stories, we are reassured we can get through our own difficulties and become better human beings.

My mother kept statues of her favorite saints in the window and even changed their outfits depending on what she was praying for. Different colors symbolized a request, promise, sorrow, or gratitude. Green was my favorite—the color of hope and of life. Certain saints were special because they were the protectors of our ancestral Italian family towns. St. Rocco, for example was the patron saint of Girifalco, a little town in the province of Catanzaro, Calabria, where my grandfather was born. Each year, the people gather to honor its patron saint, considered protector from the plague and all contagious diseases. The celebration begins with a Holy Mass, then a parade through town, punctuated by the music of local musicians, an alms-giving ceremony, and then of course a bread-breaking tradition as people come together as a community.

Most Italians share a baptismal name with a saint, so family and close friends will acknowledge each other's name day, or *onomastico*, with a greeting, a card, a little gift, or special sweets. Having your own saint assigned to you feels special and provides a personal connection with a saint who is most closely watching over you.

Here are just a few saints who are well loved in Italy:

Carlo Acutis. If you don't think saints live among us or have relevance in contemporary times, you need only look to the recent life of Italian teenager Carlo Acutis, not quite a full-fledged saint yet at the time of this writing. Acutis was beatified by the Catholic Church on October 10, 2020. With evidence of just one more miracle, he will be confirmed as the patron saint of the internet. Born in 1991, Acutis died of leukemia at age fifteen after creating a website that documented numerous Eucharistic miracles around the world. From heaven, he is said to have cured a Brazilian boy of a rare pancreatic disorder after the boy touched a piece of a T-shirt that belonged to Acutis. His example of computer skills, cheerfulness, and the dedication of his short life to helping the disadvantaged make him a role model for teens today.

St. Francis of Assisi, who lived during the Middle Ages, is considered the patron saint of Italy. He is best known for renouncing the wealth of both his family and the church and living a life of poverty to follow in the footsteps of Jesus. He had many followers and built a humble little chapel, which can be seen as a metaphor for the pure and simple life he lived, devoted to loving God and all God's creatures, especially animals. His chapel today can be found inside the Basilica di Santa Maria degli Angeli, in the town of Assisi. Through his example, we learn that having money and riches pale greatly in comparison to living a life of love and simplicity.

San Gennaro, a bishop who lived in the third century, is the adored patron saint of Naples, Italy. His blood, which is preserved in a solid state, is said to liquify three times a year: September 19 (the saint's feast day), December 16, and the first Saturday in May.

The vial containing the blood is put out for public veneration, and if it does not liquify, especially on Gennaro's feast day, it is taken as a bad omen, foreshadowing a disaster of some kind.

Padre Pio is passionately venerated by southern Italians, who consider him as one of their own for his relatability and proximity to their hometowns. Canonized in 2002 by Pope John Paul II, he is also known as St. Pius of Pietrelcina. On a wall in my home is a hand-crocheted likeness of Padre Pio, made by a cousin who lives in Castelpagano, a town not too far from the saint's hometown. During Padre Pio's priesthood, he began to notice the reappearing marks, pain, and occasional bleeding of stigmata on his hands and feet corresponding to the wounds caused by the crucifixion of Jesus Christ. These wounds were said to smell like flowers or have the aroma of sanctity. St. Pius is considered the patron saint of adolescents, stress relief, and volunteer civil defense workers.

St. Anthony of Padova. I had to smile when I recently heard a Jewish friend of mine praying to St. Anthony when she was having a hard time finding a kitchen utensil she needed for her recipe. It was the same refrain I learned as a child, and to this day, I can attest that it works! *St. Anthony, St. Anthony, please come around. Something [add the object] has been lost and has to be found.*

Fai da Te

HOW TO CONNECT WITH SAINTS

Whether you believe in saints from a religious perspective or have more of a secular curiosity about their lives, you can still find inspiration from reading about them. Here is an interesting exercise. Check to see if your first or middle name corresponds to a saint's name, and read all about that saint, noting any commonalities between their characteristics and yours. There is no shortage of encyclopedic volumes pertaining to saints. One book that many readers seem to enjoy is *The Complete Illustrated Encyclopedia of Saints*. If you were not named for a saint, then look up the saint who is associated with a special concern you are experiencing. Read about that saint's life, and reflect on the ways they overcame their challenges. List any admirable qualities of the saints you read about, and let them motivate you to develop more of those qualities in yourself.

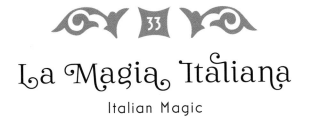

La Magia Italiana

Italian Magic

Magic is sometimes thought of as something that enchants us and lifts us temporarily out of ordinary life. The ancient Romans used magic for happiness and well-being. Their hopes, dreams, and desires were not so different from what human beings express today: health and well-being and protection from harm. We all need a little "magic" in our lives. We are drawn to the mystery of what the limitation of our senses can't verify. Italian life is described as la dolce vita not so much because of the Fellini movie but because it embraces both the supernatural and the natural. There is a seamless juxtaposition of enlightened thinking and ancient superstition, which is exhilarating and at times dizzying, as evidenced in the following ways.

Saint Worship

Italian Catholics participate in what some describe as a cult-like worship of saints in exchange for *la promessa*, the promise of good health. In southern Italy, there is still a firm belief in magic, witchcraft, folk healers, religious rituals, and over-the-top holy festivals, many of which display dramatic reenactments of biblical scenes. The sacred and the profane are often found *a braccetto* (arm in arm). Despite a contemporary, more enlightened dismissal of supernatural beliefs, some modern variations of old-world magical folk rituals are becoming increasingly popular among younger generations of Italians in recent times.

Witchcraft

At one time, Italian *stregheria* was far more widespread throughout Italy. Essentially, witches were seen as earthly beings with supernatural powers. Some were believed to be healers and able to cure illnesses. Bad witches cast spells. The two should be distinguished, but both have had a major impact on the fabric of Italian culture. *Aradia, or the Gospel of the Witches* was written in 1899 by Charles Godfrey Leland, a Princeton-educated writer and self-proclaimed folklorist. In it, he documents a mishmash of information on the origins, spells, rituals, and beliefs of pre-Etruscan pagan witches. Leland describes what he claims to have heard referred to as *la vecchia religione* (the old religion, most likely referring to the pagan deities) as something "more than sorcery" and "less than faith." The bulk of his information came from his "witch informant," whom he called "Maddalena."

When the Catholic Church eventually outlawed witchcraft, it began to fade out and be displaced by Christian elements, sometimes mixed with folk magic practices. The "Christianized" contemporary version of Italian witchcraft was born out of fear of offending God and is considered "fake" witchcraft, and according to expert Paolo Giordano (at Stregheria.com), any witchcraft that uses Christian symbols such as rosary beads or holy water is not *authentic* witchcraft. Nor does *true* witchcraft consist of old family rituals involving scissors, oil, salt, etc. The history and origins of Italian witchcraft are complex and have been continually reinterpreted and revised with the passage of time. Originally *la stregheria* was a pagan practice with an intent to do harm, perhaps to those belonging to a higher oppressive class. Later, when the Catholic Church renounced witchcraft, remnants of the original practices survived by becoming interwoven with some Christian elements, and then somewhere along the line, folk magic and folk healing practiced by those in more remote Italian villages (for example, the *malocchio*) came to be categorized by some as having elements of witchery.

Dr. Sabina Magliocco's article "Imagining the Strega" describes Italian American witchcraft as a "folklore reclamation" that attempts to revive the folklore practices of the Italian immigrants who came to America at the turn of the century but whose practices at that time were marginalized by the dominant culture. The elements of their practices were reinterpreted and adopted as symbols of identity and pride generations later. On the other hand, these practices have also caused Italian Americans to be the brunt of jokes and stereotyping.

My father's family comes from a little province of Benevento, a city where—legend has it—a walnut tree sat along the banks of the Sabato River where the Romans were said to have performed pagan rituals to worship the Egyptian goddess Isis, and eventually witches were said to fly in to the *noce* (nut tree) each year to cast evil spells, then fly off again. *Le streghe* also brewed a powerful love potion in their cauldron, which united lovers forever if drunk. In 1860, the golden liqueur called Strega was created in Benevento, containing saffron and over seventy herbs and spices from all over the world. There was always a bottle of Strega in my grandmother's cabinet, which would be brought out when company came. Most Italian Catholics—even if not considered practicing Catholics—will have some recollection, as I do, of our parents putting garlic around our necks during flu season, putting religious statues in the window to influence the weather, or having their grandmother perform the *malocchio* ritual.

La smorfia napoletana

Named for Morpheus, the god of dreams in Greek mythology, this is the Neapolitan (or Italian) dream dictionary corresponding to lottery numbers. My grandmother would often mention a dream she had, and the symbols or words in the dream would translate to a number, which she was certain should be played in the current lottery. Some examples include Italy = 1, baby = 2, cat = 3, pig = 4, hand = 5, etc.

Tarantism

While we may dance the tarantella at Italian weddings, the ritual of the *taranta*, or trance dancing, is often associated with Puglia and Sardegna. Reportedly when an insect or spider bite caused the victim (usually a woman working out in the fields) to become possessed by the arachnid's (*tarantola*) spirit, she would develop symptoms that could include anything from headaches to convulsions. Special musicians who knew how to match the fast-paced rhythm of the spider and connect with the personality of the afflicted with their tambourine, accordion, flute, and/or guitars would be called, and the bite victim would dance for hours, even days, until the bite was exorcised.

Today in Italy, while many experts in the fields of anthropology and psychology don't necessarily believe to the letter in the classic tarantism cure, they do feel that the dancing was a type of movement that freed nervous energy from the body and did have some value. We know that dance changes our mood and lifts our spirits. A form of the tarantella dance, sometimes called the *pizzica*, is danced throughout Italy's town squares at festivals and events.

Amulets

Do you wear an amulet for good luck or do you wear one to keep the evil spirits at bay? Many Italians do, whether they actually believe in superstition or not—just to be on the safe side. Going back to ancient Roman times, symbols of fertility, like the phallus, were supposed to bring good luck. Fish, snakes, even keys in the folk vernacular are metaphors for the penis and often found in amulets.

The *corno* or horn, representing the virile ram, is one that everyone knows. You will see gaudy red plastic horns in souvenir shops now, but they were originally made from rich red Mediterranean coral. The *mano cornuta*—or horned hand—is a fist with the pointer and little fingers pointing out. I have one in gold, but it is also a gesture that wards off the evil eye and can be made from gold or silver.

Rue (*Ruta graveolens*) is a medicinal herb frequently used by folk healers to treat a number of ailments as well as protect against the evil eye. As an amulet, it is called a *cimaruta*, typically made in silver, and it looks like a lacy sprig and goes back to ancient Etruscan and Roman times when the *cimaruta* was also hung over a baby's bed to ward off the evil eye. *Mano fica*—also a fertility symbol—protects against the evil eye and is represented by a closed fist over a thumb whose tip juts out between the pointer and middle finger.

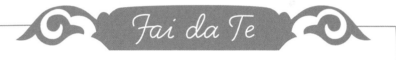

Fai da Te

ADD AN AMULET TO YOUR JEWELRY COLLECTION

You don't have to believe in the supernatural or in rituals or talismans to have fun with Italian magic. A dolce vita perspective embraces opposites as natural and peacefully coexisting. Even if you want to just be "on the safe side" or want a cool piece of jewelry that can also serve as a conversation starter, do a search of online jewelry catalogues for Italian amulets. For less expensive options, you will also see a variety of traditional Italian charms on Amazon, Etsy, or websites like GrandVoyageItaly.com.

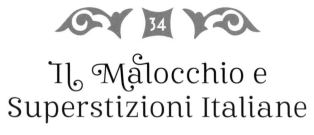

Il Malocchio e Superstizioni Italiane

The Evil Eye and Other Italian Superstitions

Italy is often described as a culture of contradiction, where superstition and religiosity coexist peacefully. Recent studies on magical thinking and superstition, as opposed to previous beliefs, have confirmed that people who believe in superstition and rituals to protect themselves from those beliefs are neither cognitively deficient nor necessarily experiencing some form of psychopathology. That's a relief to those Italians who still follow rituals, such as the *malocchio* (evil eye), to guard against bad luck—even if they don't *really* believe in them. Some will say it is ridiculous to believe in ancient superstition, but if you totally dismiss it, you may have bad luck!

Ancient folklore, healing rituals, superstition, and remedies not only provide an interesting look into a culture's past, but some people choose to incorporate such rituals in a secular spiritual practice as a way of honoring their ancestors. "Ancestral veneration," as it is called, is a way of honoring the memory of those who came before us, because if not for them, we would not exist. Occasionally spiritual home altars may be dedicated to deceased predecessors. Nonspiritual ways of honoring our ancestors include doing genealogical research; learning about their lifestyles, superstitions, rituals, music, and recipes; or learning what dances they did. Even pouring over old photographs of the loved ones in your past can bring a feeling of wonder and well-being. All these processes are said to keep the energy of our loved ones alive as well as maintain our bonds with them. While learning about and honoring our ancestors can provide the comfort of belonging through a salient connection to our roots, perhaps the greatest way we could have pleased them is to fulfill our highest potential and live a happy life.

Italian Superstitions

Some common Italian superstitions involve numbers. The number thirteen, for example, is lucky, while Friday the seventeenth is so unlucky that many hotels don't even mark a seventeenth floor. This belief can be traced back to ancient Roman times when one anagram of the Roman number XVII signified that life was over.

Hats, in Italy, are never left on the bed. In the old days when a priest came to anoint the dying, he would take off his hat and place it on the bed. Placing one's hat on the bed even today is seen as an omen for impending death.

Spilling salt or olive oil can also bring bad luck, as can opening an umbrella inside the home, toasting with water instead of wine in your glass, or breaking a mirror. Italians will go the extra mile to protect themselves from bad energy by touching iron or saying "*tocca ferro*" (similar to our "knock on wood") to ensure nothing they said might attract misfortune. They might also carry or wear an amulet (such as a horn-shaped coral charm), wear a coral horn on a chain, or make a fist with protruding index and pinkie finger in the shape of horns.

In southern Italy, people used to believe that someone can intentionally or unintentionally cause harm to another—either physically or emotionally—just by looking at them a certain way or complimenting them a little too much. This is what is known as *il malocchio*, or the "evil eye." If someone compliments you on your appearance or property or makes a fuss over the baby you are pushing in a stroller, it might be taken as a sign of envy,

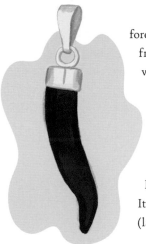

foretelling that something likely will be taken away from you as a result. Either a knowledgeable older woman, the grandmother of the family, or a *strega* (witch) would know how to dispel the *malocchio* by performing a certain ritual while reciting a prayer. While the rituals varied from village to village, the basic remedy for the *malocchio* was documented by the Rhode Island Folklife Project, with archived photographs of Italian women removing the spell of the *malocchio* (labeled under the category "Italian traditions").

To do this, one would take a small bowl of water and a spoonful of olive oil. The sign of the cross is made over the spoon of olive oil and over the bowl of water while a silent prayer is spoken, naming the person who is suspected of having been cursed by the *malocchio*. Five drops of oil are dropped into the water from the spoon, using the little finger for each drop. If the oil disperses on the water instead of staying together in droplets, it is assumed that the person named has *malocchio*. This ritual is repeated three times to remove the spell.

The Paranormal

One of the most influential mediums of the late nineteenth and early twentieth centuries was a middle-aged Italian woman whom some referred to as the diva of the supernatural, Eusapia Palladino (1854–1918). Palladino, who was born of humble beginnings in a province of Bari, went from being an uneducated and illiterate orphan child to eventually being sought after by the wealthiest and most prestigious members of the international scene, including Broadway stars such as Grace George and William A. Brady, Nobel Prize laureates Marie and Pierre Curie, and world-renowned Italian psychiatrist and criminologist Cesare Lombroso. Attendees around her séance table swore they saw and heard her contact the dead. Palladino's managers booked her séances in her native Italy, England, France, Poland, Russia, Germany, and the United States. News accounts spread with tabloid sensationalism by witnesses who said they saw tables levitating, objects moving, curtains waving, body parts materializing, and lights flashing when the entranced Palladino channeled her spirit guide "John King." Palladino was quite convincing. Even today, over one hundred years later, her history of deception is still sometimes brushed aside by those who write and teach about her.

Eusapia Palladino was caught using trickery throughout her career and even admitted to it. Yet blind credulity, even among some respected behavioral scientists, would continue to persist. Ultimately, the American branch of the Society for Psychic Research demonstrated conclusively that her powers were due to trickery, such as making her sitters believe she was touching them with both hands when she was really only touching them with one. She achieved this by slowly moving together the hands of the sitters on either side of her and sliding her own hand out of the "chain." The objects that moved across the table during her séances had been pulled with a hair, which of course could not be seen in the dark. Palladino's own hand or foot would cause a curtain to move, and so on.

While up to this point science has not been able to prove or disprove whether those who call themselves mediums can really communicate with the dead, for some people who are grieving, mediums provide a message that can offer a bit of happiness or, at the very least, tranquility in hearing that a loved one is okay and watching over them.

Fai da Te

DO YOUR HOMEWORK BEFORE PAYING A PSYCHIC

Ultimately, our beliefs are personal, and no one has the right to judge another for believing or not in the world of psychics or in the veracity of a séance. Psychic readings may provide comfort to some, but for others, they might disappoint. Here are some tips you might find useful.

* Know what you want to get out of a session with a medium. You might feel a weight lifted from your shoulders just hearing someone tell you that your loved one forgives you or that they are proud of what you have become. On the other hand, you might feel cheated out of your hard-earned dollars if you don't at least come out with more specific information.

* Since there are currently no controlled laboratory studies that prove psychic mediums are actually communicating with the dead, look to online reviews or word of mouth from people you know who have been satisfied with that person.

* Ask ahead of time what the fees are and what you can reasonably expect for your session.

* Consider hiring a psychic or medium not to talk to your deceased loved ones or to predict your future but, like many people today, allow them to serve as your happiness coach, teaching you how to tune in to your own instinctual awareness and inner guide.

35

L'Arte di Arrangiarsi

The Art of Getting By

I recently watched an interview with distinguished Italian philosopher, academic, and psychoanalyst Umberto Galimberti. He was addressing the question: How do you get back up when life beats you down? When you experience grief, depression, sadness, or other major life challenges? The remedy is to act, not to stay still. Do something—anything. Take action. Get a job at an ice cream shop, volunteer on a farm, take a long walk—anything that causes you to act. In other words, keep moving.

We know from research that physical activity, including exercise, can turn a sad mood around, but it is also not dissimilar to what Italians refer to as *l'arte di arrangiarsi*, which loosely translated implies that you do the best you can to get by in a difficult situation. Often, even starting with the simple step of getting to your feet and taking a walk around the block can be the catalyst for an important turning point. Doing what you have to do to move forward does not mean lying in bed, fantasizing about what could have been, or curling up into a ball and giving up. It is about accepting the reality of the situation and then doing something to move through the difficulty.

Maybe there is something you can change about the problematic situation itself, or if not, you can certainly change your perspective on it. Pairing problem-solving strategies with actual physical movement to improve your mood can help you feel more in control of your situation and your emotions.

In addition to being a possible *remedy* for sadness, physical activity has also been found to possibly *prevent* depression.

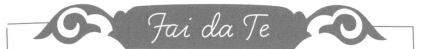

Fai da Te

PRACTICE THE ITALIAN ART OF GETTING
BY WHEN TIMES GET TOUGH

Rest assured that by virtue of being human we have the inner strength to handle any situation that happens to human beings. Find support when you need it, but above all never stop believing in yourself when life's challenges arise. Here are some ideas:

❀ Tell yourself that you will not let bad situations defeat you. Positive self-talk is empowering.

❀ Get up on your feet, get out the door, and **do** something. Take a walk, cut the lawn, volunteer, take on a part-time job, go dancing, wash your car, water your plants, or engage in any other activity that involves physically moving your body.

❀ Do the best you can when life gets tough. You don't have to be perfect or do everything right. Brainstorm ways in which you might change the actual situation itself or how to think differently about it if the situation is unchangeable. Learn to accept reality, and continue to live your life with determination and gratitude.

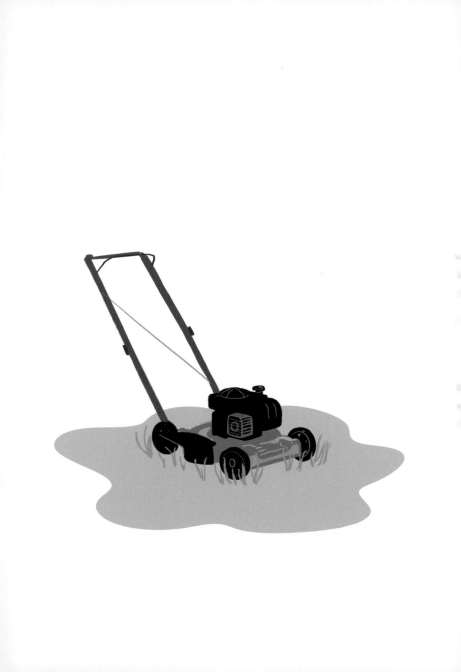

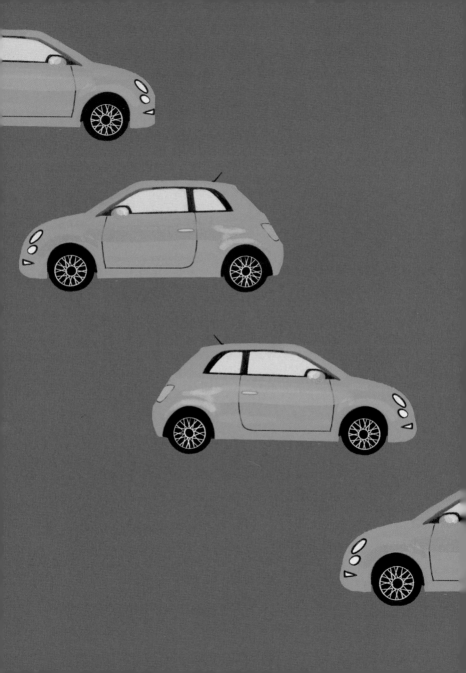

The Italian Celebration of Lifestyle

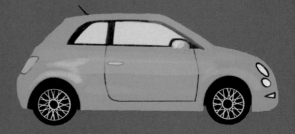

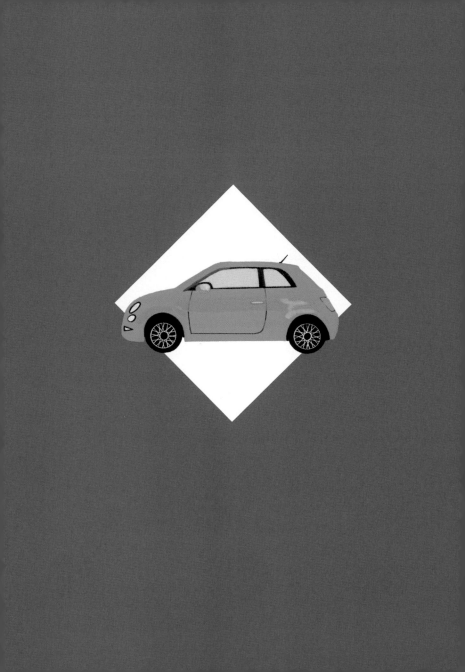

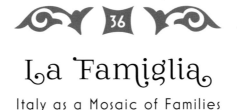

La Famiglia

Italy as a Mosaic of Families

The strength of Italy lies in the strength of its *famiglie*. Luigi Barzini, in his classic book *The Italians*, described Italy as a "mosaic of families who stick together instinctually like ants." In a zeitgeist that is sometimes harsh, with political and religious institutions that are not always trusted, there is one unit that will always supply protection, comfort, and insulation as well as take care of every need of its individual members—*la famiglia*, the Italian family.

Years ago, the Italian family unit was large and self-sufficient. A lot of children meant a lot of hands to work the farm, maintain the house, or help run the family business. Generations would live together in one big house; sons brought their wives to live with their family of origin after marriage. If you needed anything—money, car repair, help to harvest the grapes or build an addition to your house, someone to babysit or stay with a sick or elderly member—someone in the family or extended family would pool together to take care of it. Family stuck together. The traditional Italian family was patriarchal; the father figure provided financial support, and the mother tended to the home and the education of the children as well as arranging for the family's social life.

Today, that classic family structure has changed, as women have made headway into the workplace. The Italian birth rate has also dropped, and on average, families now have a single child per couple, if that. Families are split up more than ever as younger generations move away for work opportunities. In modern times, Italian families, instead of getting together most days for dinner, will at least make it a point to be together for special festivities and holidays. The familial bond, however, is rarely broken nor typically weakened by estrangement between generations.

The *famiglia* is a source of strength and learning. It is how children learn manners and skills; how to wash, clean, and build; and how to be in the world. It is where one learns how to trust, how to grow a thick skin, how to manage relationships, and how to let go. The media likes to sensationalize Italian family loyalty by framing it within the context of organized crime, but loyalty is the unspoken code of *every* Italian family, the majority of whom have nothing at all to do with organized crime and abhor it just as much as anyone else does. Italian parents still carefully guard their family privacy and teach children from a young age that what goes on in the family stays within the walls of the family home.

Family relationships—both positive and negative—have been shown to have a significant impact on personal well-being throughout our lives. Supportive family relationships foster greater self-esteem, self-confidence, optimism, positive emotions, better coping skills, and in general better mental health. Italian families respect their elders and treat children like royalty. Children are allowed to be children even if they are dressed well and never leave home without their faces washed. There will be time enough to learn to do chores, but childhood is a magical time that should be filled with play and exploration and smothered with kisses.

Generational wisdom within Italian families is not to be taken for granted. Marcus Aurelius began his book of meditations with an homage to the members of his family to whom he was forever grateful for what they taught him about life. From his grandfather, Aurelius learned good morals and ways to control his temper. From his mother, he learned how to live simply and piously. From his great-grandfather, he learned to have good teachers at home. From his brother, he learned how to love his kin and to practice truth and justice.

Everyone has a special role in the Italian family, but perhaps the central role is that of *la mamma*. An Italian proverb states, "*Una buona mamma vale cento maestre*" (A good mother is worth a hundred teachers). One of the most famous Italian ballads is not directed to the singer's lover but rather to his mother. The term *mammone* refers to the close bond that Italian men usually have with their mothers for life. The classic 1940 Italian song "Mamma" never fails to make Italians weep from the nostalgia of days gone by, being cared for by their loving mother. The song has been sung by everyone from Luciano Pavarotti to Jerry Vale to Frank Sinatra to Il Volo.

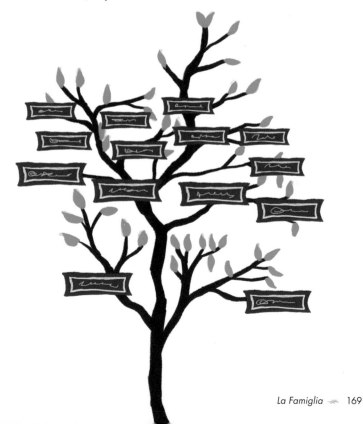

Fai da Te

REFLECT ON THE WISDOM OF YOUR FAMILY

Not every family relationship is supportive, yet we learn valuable life lessons and hopefully important coping skills if we are lucky. Here is an exercise that might help put your family dynamics into perspective and let you recognize how each relationship allowed you to evolve and develop into the beautiful human being you are.

In a little notebook, list all the life lessons you have learned (you can keep adding to it) through the example or advice of each member of your family, past and present. Include extended family members—even family members you don't care for (we cannot choose our family). We learn something from every familial relationship.

This exercise provides a perfect opportunity to get in touch with relatives you haven't connected with in a while. Invite them for coffee, have a long telephone chat, or send them a thoughtful card in the mail. Bring your family closer if possible by organizing regular get-togethers. If you have no blood relatives (or for good reason prefer not to interact with them), consider close friends as honorary family members.

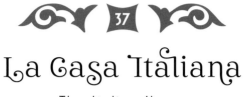

La Casa Italiana

The Italian Home

To get an idea of how your surroundings affect your mood, imagine it is a hot summer day. You find yourself sitting in a landfill, with trash and junk everywhere. The stench is making you nauseous. Seagulls are soaring overhead to scavenge whatever they can find and leaving their droppings all around you; flies are buzzing around to get their fill too, occasionally landing on your skin until you swipe them away. An occasional rodent runs for cover under a mound of garbage. Most likely your mood is not cheery. Quite the contrary, you might feel bummed out, repulsed, frustrated by all the "ugliness."

Now imagine it is a crisp, cool day and you are sitting at the edge of a tall mountain. You look out into a clear turquoise sky decorated with cotton clouds that float slowly by in the gentle breeze. The panorama is expansive and breathtaking. You feel lucky to be alive. You feel invigorated and grateful. You may even have a sense of the spiritual.

As discussed earlier, beauty matters. Dr. Piero Ferrucci, in his book *Beauty and the Soul*, wrote that "beauty is a factor that stimulates our joy of living." Human beings have an aesthetic intelligence. The positive feelings beauty elicits in us last long after the experience. Nature is the ultimate architect of beauty, but we are the architects of the beauty that surrounds our living spaces. Italians, regardless of financial status, take great pains to make their homes neat, clean, and attractive.

Whether you prefer a Tuscan rustic interior, an art-centric Renaissance décor, or an ornate baroque-style home, Italians follow two basic house-related principles:

 1   The home should be well organized.

2   Cleanliness is next to godliness.

Cleaning is a passion in the *bel paese*, and having a clean, organized home gives a satisfied feeling of accomplishment.

According to a survey Procter & Gamble conducted some years ago, Italians spend at least twenty-one hours per week on household chores as compared to four hours for Americans. They also purchase more cleaning supplies than do people in most other countries, according to survey data, and they prefer the cleaning process to be slow and thorough rather than done with quick and easy shortcuts. No lick and a scrub here. Bathroom floors are washed and scrubbed at least four times a week (often with a combination of mop and elbow grease on one's hands and knees), which accounts for why those marble, slate, or terrazzo floors look like squared mirrored plates you could eat off. Also, forget taking your shoes off before entering an Italian home, as cleaning the floor every day is a given and more preferable than seeing (or smelling) a visitor's bare feet!

Some Interesting Tidbits about Italian Homes

Air-conditioning is not usually found in Italian homes. Italians have a fear (if not phobia) of drafts and catching a chill. Growing up, we were never allowed to leave the house with wet or damp hair, nor to sit near an open window if there was a breeze coming through. Italians are also energy conscious and prefer to open windows and use fans to keep air circulating through their homes.

A balcony is an important part of the Italian apartment. From *Romeo and Juliet* to the pope delivering his blessing to the people to the COVID-19

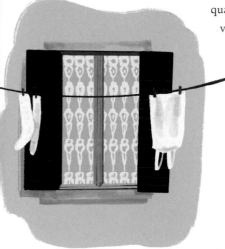

quarantine, the balcony inspires and provides a way to keep connected to others (as seen in news clips of Italians singing, playing instruments, launching fireworks, and—more recently—applauding healthcare workers). The balcony provides sunlight and fresh air for the first cup of morning coffee, for the plants that embellish it, and for the laundry that gently flaps and dances in the breeze that floats across it.

Window coverings or curtains are important for privacy. Italians' windows are heavy for insulation and open up wide to the sides, as do the shutters that protect them. Curtains keep people on the outside from looking inside your home, which is also a good safety measure.

Italian toilets, or *water* (pronounced "vater"), are not water-filled bowls but rather holes, allowing waste to slide directly down and out of sight. Then, to make sure one's bottom is clean, almost every home (and hotel) in Italy has a bidet, which is like a toilet-shaped sink of sorts, allowing you to wash your bottom whenever you want to feel clean without having to take an entire shower.

Rather than making up one's bed immediately upon waking, many Italians like to turn down the bedding, open the window, and let the bed "air out." Fresh air is welcomed throughout the home when the weather permits.

The process of cleaning can feel therapeutic. That is how it was for the Italian women in my family. They were particular about what products and machines they used (or avoided). Many Italian women iron nearly all the laundry—including sheets and socks. While you don't have to go quite that far, there is something to be said for immersing yourself in the meditative rhythm of cleaning house. No matter how modest or fancy, an Italian home is a thing of beauty because of the way it is lovingly maintained.

A clean and organized home lends itself to a happy atmosphere. Make a daily and weekly house cleaning and organization plan to keep yourself on track and avoid becoming so overwhelmed that you lose motivation and don't know where to start. Don't think of cleaning as an unpleasant experience to avoid. Be fully present during every step of the process, and notice how a clean and organized home gives you great satisfaction.

Fai da Te

CONSIDER NATURAL ITALIAN CLEANING SOLUTIONS

Before the advent of commercial chemically manufactured products, it was common to use natural products to clean house. That tradition is making a comeback among Italians. White vinegar and hot water make an excellent combination for washing floors, cleaning up grease splatters on stove tops, and removing fingerprints from large kitchen appliances. Wipe surfaces with a dry, soft cloth for a nice shine. A bit of baking soda added to the mixture makes an effective toilet, sink, and tub scrub. Make sure to rinse thoroughly with water. Lemon oil makes a nontoxic furniture polish. Common dish or castile soap can help with spots on carpets.

An article published once in *Donna Moderna*, one of Italy's most popular magazines, mentioned *sapone di Marsiglia* (Marseille soap) as a staple in many Italian households. It is a very pure, mild soap that comes in powder, solid, or liquid form. The liquid soap can be used for a myriad of cleaning tasks, and you can easily purchase it online (e.g., Amazon) even if you don't live in Italy.

Also, keep a few bottles of essential oils in your cleaning arsenal to add a fresh scent to the natural cleaning agents. Some dolce vita favorites include natural lavender, tea tree oil, and citrus. Fresh lemons, white vinegar, baking soda, and borax pretty much complete your main cleaning ingredients. Various combinations of these few substances will clean just about anything you want to make sparkle, and you don't have to wear a mask to use them.

Donna Moderna reminds us that an old toothbrush dipped in a paste of baking soda mixed with a few drops of water works great for cleaning in between bathroom tile cracks or tight floor corners. Drains can be unclogged with boiling water to which a spoonful of cream of tartar, baking soda, and salt have been added. You can make a do-it-yourself degreaser by filling an empty spray bottle with a splash of white vinegar or lemon juice added to hot water. Add a drop of essential oil for a nice scent. Spray this on windows and mirrors, and wipe dry with old newspapers. Nonna always reminded us never to clean the windows when the sun is shining brightly, as it may leave streaks.

How to clean your bathroom? Pour some baking soda and a splash of white vinegar into the toilet bowl; then brush as usual. For surfaces, add some borax to water with a drop of essential oil; then use either as a spray or dip a sponge in the mixture and wring it out. Floors can be washed with a bucket of hot water and a few drops of *sapone di Marsiglia*. Lavender or pine essential oil adds some freshness. Make sure to dry your floor after damp mopping with some old towels or sheets.

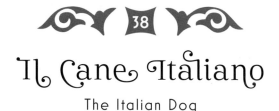

Il Cane Italiano

The Italian Dog

There is no debate regarding the emotional and physical benefits of having a pet to care for. Several scholarly articles show that having a dog or cat can reduce stress, anxiety, and depression, alleviate loneliness, and improve cardiovascular health by encouraging exercise. We all love our pets, but many tourists to the *bel paese* have posed this question: What is it about Italian dogs that makes them seem so much more serene than dogs in the United States or other countries? Why do statistics still show a far lower percentage of dog bites, dog fights, and dog maulings in Italy (and in Europe in general) than in the United States?

Some say it is because dogs in Italy are considered more of a natural element of daily life—nothing more and nothing less. You will often see Italian dogs—even unleashed—paying no attention to strangers but rather walking or sitting calmly alongside their owner. Just being an unobtrusive part of the daily social scene is all that is necessary for a harmonious cohabitation. In Italy, dogs are also allowed in more places than just pet food stores. They are rarely if ever caged in a crate all day (in some European countries, crates are actually illegal and only allowed to be used for transportation or when a dog is recovering from surgery). Italian mothers do not encourage their children to pet strange dogs, nor are dog owners who run into each other along the cobblestone streets commonly asking if their dogs could meet and sniff each other out. Dogs are not treated as entertainment in Italy, nor given sharp commands one moment and high-pitched baby talk the next. From self-reported data, it is clear that Italians, like Americans, consider their pet canines to be important family members—just not necessarily *human* family members. Perhaps therein lies an important distinction. And let's face it: Italy has a lot more experience cohabiting with our canine companions than we do.

Dogs have played an important role across the European continent as early as the Roman Empire. From archaeological examinations in Pompeii, a city that was buried and destroyed by the violent Vesuvius volcano of 79 AD, researchers have found evidence of intentional breeding of dogs for different purposes. Smaller dogs, for example, were valued as companions, while larger dogs were used to hunt with or to guard homes, as we learned from the tragic plaster cast of the Pompeian guard dog left chained to his post to be suffocated by the rising ash of the volcano.

Today, according to a 2021 ISTAT survey, about 25 percent of households in Italy include a dog (that number jumped up by 18 percent in the previous year alone, according to the most recent report from Statista), and a little under 20 percent of Italian households include cats. Love for animals can be found everywhere along the Italian peninsula. A few cases in point:

❉ Approximately 82 percent of Italians, according to a market research group, consider their pets to be actual members of the family.

❉ Pope Francis once scolded young Italian couples for preferring having pets over having children!

❁ Roman mayor Roberto Gualtieri once called for a New Year's Eve firework ban, not only to protect human safety and avoid polluting the environment but also to avoid frightening animals.

❁ Rome has its own designated beach for dogs. Located near Fiumicino Airport, Baubeach has been in operation for twenty-three years. Well-behaved dogs are free to play, swim, and run unleashed while owners can take a yoga class if they wish.

❁ An IKEA in Italy welcomed stray dogs that needed food and a place to sleep.

It's been said that perhaps Italians interact with their dogs the way Americans interact with our service dogs. When service dogs are with their owner, they are allowed to just be in order to give their full attention to their owner and avoid being distracted. They are not to be touched by strangers, made to do tricks for our entertainment, nor will you see them dressed up in cutesy uncomfortable costumes for the sake of making a human smile. Seeing their loyal and adoring face each day is all we should ever need. But dogs are more than just a cute face to look at. They have been shown to decrease loneliness, increase socialization, reduce stress and negative emotions, and give us a sense of purpose in caring for another living being.

Fai da Te

BRING A PET INTO YOUR LIFE

Italians aren't the only ones who love their pets. Most of us do. If you already have a pet, make sure you not only feed, walk, water, and groom it but also remember that they love to be talked to, sung to, and played with. Bring your furry family member to as many places as allowed to desensitize them to new and strange experiences.

If you don't have the kind of lifestyle that is conducive to owning a dog or cat, you can volunteer to walk and play with the dogs at your local animal shelter; donate pet food, blankets, toys, leashes, harnesses, and collars to them; or donate to an organization that works to protect our animals and ensures they have good-quality lives. In Italy, it is understood that our animals are special creatures. They give us joy and remind us that all species are connected through our love.

39

I Piccoli Piaceri

The Small Pleasures

One day, while visiting with my family in Italy, we had just finished the most exquisite *cena fatta in casa* (homemade supper) when out comes a bowl of juicy ripe *nespole*, or Italian loquat fruit, which is kind of a cross between a peach and an apricot. Introduced to Italy in the eighteenth century, these exquisite orange-colored ovals were once believed to have magical powers, and frankly, I could believe it. They were so scrumptious and nothing like I had ever tasted. When I mentioned to my relatives that I had never tasted a *nespola*, they immediately began pointing out details—with no lack of enthusiasm—on how to plant them and how I might grow them myself when I got back to the States. Before I knew it, everyone began cleaning off their large *nespole* pits and collecting them in a bag for me to take with me back home, along with instructions, so that I may have this tasty Italian fruit whenever I wanted it from my own backyard. Such a mundane thing as watching me enjoy their fruit turned into an impromptu point of celebration that evening and the highlight of our entire visit together. This happens all the time in the treasured land of my ancestors, who always somehow manage to elevate the ordinary to the extraordinary.

The words *dolce vita* are not just meant to be a random set of letters plastered on a restaurant sign or a travel agency website. The real Italian dolce vita, or sweet life, is the ability to let ourselves be awed by ordinary everyday pleasures that we typically don't even notice. We all have the ability to live with this sense of wonder.

I piccoli piaceri (simple pleasures) for Italians might include taking the time to pay tribute to the colors of a rainbow, like that colleague of mine from Parma who once stopped traffic at a four-way intersection to get out of his car and hoist himself up a pole to get a better look. It could be a Sunday afternoon picnic of thick crusty bread, ripe tomatoes, a wedge of cheese, fruit, and a bottle of local wine, enjoyed beneath the shade of a chestnut tree. Sitting at an outdoor café and observing passersby, making a tiramisu with friends, enjoying a rich espresso, or wrapping yourself up in the comfort of a shawl your grandmother once knitted for you—all these things (and I know you can name a thousand more) are the small daily pleasures that make Italian life so satisfying. Savoring small pleasures is at the heart of Italian dolce vita. These are the things we often fail to notice while in the throes of our busy routines.

When I was a college professor, I once gave my students the assignment of describing the details of the corridor floors they had just walked across on their way into my classroom. I would estimate that less than 10 percent of the class was able to recall with complete accuracy the design and color of the flooring, even though they walked that same floor day after day over the course of the semester—and had just walked over it right before our class began! Frankly, if I hadn't carried out that exercise as part of a unit on attention and memory, I probably would never have been able to recall the details of the hallway floor myself. I never gave it my attention.

Because our cognitive resources have limits, the human tendency is to pay more attention to what we consider the necessary things we have to get done in the course of a day while the "insignificant" stimuli go unnoticed. The cost of doing so is that we miss the many smaller detailed delights that go unnoticed. Italians seem to have pleasure-seeking radar, and they don't have to be hit over the head to notice them.

Leonardo da Vinci's keen observational skills were the tools that allowed his insatiable curiosity to appreciate even the finest detail. To represent people and nature so realistically in his art, he had to notice every feature with equal voraciousness. In his notebooks, Leonardo advised "as you go through the fields, turn your attention to various objects, and in turn, look now at this thing and now at that."

Admittedly a university floor might not be particularly worthy of attention. Likewise the ancient cobblestone alleyways throughout Rome might not give us goose bumps if we are fixated only on getting to the Colosseum, the Spanish Steps, or the Trevi Fountain. Yet if we make a point to notice details, it might elicit a surprising sense of pride to realize we are walking the same university corridors as others before us who have made an impact on the world. We might get chills of delight to think our footsteps are tracing over the same ancient cobblestones that the Romans built centuries ago in the history of mankind.

Happiness doesn't come only from momentous events or expensive possessions. Delighting in the details of an ordinary day will make every day special, and it doesn't cost a thing.

I recently read the obituary of an Italian immigrant who came to the United States to raise a family and give his kids every opportunity to reach their fullest potential. What moved me most in reading about his life were the aspects his family thought important enough to include to sum up the existence of this seemingly ordinary yet extraordinary human being. "He worked very hard to give his children a beautiful life," the tribute said, "and he enjoyed the simple pleasures of tending to his garden, cooking, and drinking espresso."

This goes to the core of what la dolce vita means to Italians.

Fai da Te

NOTICE THE LITTLE PLEASURES

Carry with you a pocket-sized notebook, and jot down all the small pleasures throughout your day. The more you make it a point to notice your blessings, the greater will be your appreciation, and you will sharpen your own Italian pleasure-seeking radar. Today you might have heard a funny story that brought tears of laughter to your eyes. Perhaps your son, daughter, or grandchild made you a birthday card or invited you to kick around a soccer ball with them. Maybe your hairdresser got the cut just right this time and you fall in love with what you see in the mirror. As you took your daily walk, you noticed a giant pink peony in your neighbor's front yard. Notice these things. Be more attentive to discovering your own treasure trove of small daily pleasures, and notice how quickly your whole life becomes far more dolce.

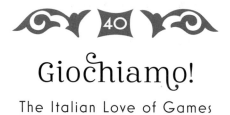

Giochiamo!

The Italian Love of Games

What do bocce (Italian version of bowling), *briscola* (a card game), *tombola* (Italian bingo), *calcio* (soccer), and the videogame *F1* (based on the Formula 1 and Formula 2 international race car championships) have in common? They are all testaments to a culture's enthusiasm for having fun. After all, an important ingredient of the dolce vita is balance. Work hard when you are at work; enjoy fun and laughter when you're not. As it turns out, making time for fun activities actually improves mood and promotes well-being. "Pleasant activity scheduling," as it is referred to in the psychology journals, is sometimes used as a therapeutic technique to reduce stress, banish a negative mood, and increase happiness. Social get-togethers for the sole purpose of playing a game, orchestrating a sing-along, or even cheering at a televised sports event are in Italy's cultural DNA.

Most of us, however, don't schedule pleasant activities as part of our regular week. We think of it as a waste of time when we could be doing something more "productive," like working a few extra hours or getting chores done around the house. We say there simply are not enough hours in a day. Well, what if I could show you that there *is* a way to find time to make social playtime a priority? It is called the Pareto principle, and it can help you free up some space in your schedule to do the things you might have thought you didn't have time for.

In the late 1800s, Italian economist and mathematician Vilfredo Pareto observed that 20 percent of the people owned 80 percent of the land in Italy. More generally, the Pareto principle states that 80 percent of the consequences in most areas of life come from 20 percent of the causes. If you own a small business, for example, you might notice that 80 percent of your sales come from 20 percent of the products in your inventory. The obvious thing to do would be to either direct your marketing efforts to those top-selling items or increase inventory of similar items and eliminate what doesn't move your business forward.

The Pareto principle (often called the 80/20 rule) was eventually observed to be true in most areas of life, including personal time management. If you examine how much time you spend working on a computer, you are likely to find that 20 percent of your time actually went to getting your official work task accomplished, and 80 percent of your time online was distraction. Similarly, time management experts believe we can be much more effective—and less frazzled—if we focus our efforts on accomplishing the 20 percent of the tasks on our to-do list that are top priority, those that will really make a qualitative difference in our lives. The rest we can probably delegate or let go.

Too much busyness drains our emotional and physical resources, energy that could be funneled into increasing our happiness. Some of my best childhood memories are of the laughter arising from the nearby bocce court where my father and his friends played for hours in the summer evenings. I can still smell the coffee percolating and the biscotti baking when my mother invited friends over for an evening of card games, or my grandmother, *zio*, and I would sit around her kitchen table with a small glass of homemade wine, a plate of cheese, salami, and her *pane fatto in casa* (homemade bread) while she dealt from a special Italian deck of cards for *scopa*.

The instinct for play cuts across all cultural and time boundaries. Animals as well as humans have engaged in some kind of game playing since the beginning of time. Throwing a ball to reach a target, for instance, is an idea that can be traced back to early Egyptian society. The Egyptians came up with a template for what was later known as bocce around 5,000 BC. The ancient Romans used coconuts brought back from Africa as bocce balls. Even Galileo sung the praises of this lively game as toning the body and rejuvenating the spirit.

Calcio fiorentino (Florentine soccer) was played from the fifteenth to the eighteenth century, primarily by the upper classes in Renaissance Florence. It was a more primitive and aggressive (i.e., violent) form of the *calcio* that Italians are obsessed with today. Yet even though all-out fights would break out on the Piazza Santa Croce as teams came up against each other, *la bella figura* still mattered. Players were expected to be graceful and well dressed. In that same spirit, Italy's national team today dons uniforms designed by Giorgio Armani. From *bambini* to *nonni* and everyone in between, rarely will you find an Italian who can pass up a good game of soccer, whether scrimmaging with friends in a small town piazza or following a televised game at a neighborhood sports bar. If in the United States, the first thing one might ask when making a new acquaintance might be "What do you do for a living?" in *Italia*, the more urgent question would be "*Di che squadra sei?*" (What team do you root for?). Sports offer camaraderie, friendship, and lightheartedness. Games will be talked about, argued about, cheered about for a long time afterward, all in good fun.

Playing video games is another way Italians like to unwind. Their usage went up during the pandemic from eight to eight and a half hours a week during the first lockdown. According to Marco Saletta, chair of the Italian Interactive Digital

Entertainment Association, 38 percent of Italy's population between the ages of six and sixty-four plays video games regularly. But they don't use it to avoid interaction with others; quite the contrary. Italians used video games more during the lockdown as a way to stay *connected* to others online, when they were not able to leave their homes and socialize in person. Games can also be a way to have fun together as a family.

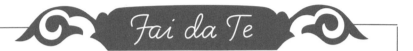

Fai da Te

LEARN AN ITALIAN GAME

One way to have more fun in your life: consider the world of games. You can choose from games that require physical skill (bocce, soccer, or volleyball), games that require chance (tombola or Italian bingo), or games that require mental strategy (card games such as *scopa* or *briscola*). Spectator sports too, when watched in good company, can help us turn off life's worries, have some laughs, and regroup before getting back to the daily routine.

If you want to find more of a balance in your day and feel like a carefree kid again, play! Schedule a regular game night with friends or family at your home. Guests can bring their favorite snack to share, or you can make an inexpensive antipasto and serve with slices of crusty bread and wine or sparkling water for those who don't drink alcohol. Rotate the choice of games, and if you don't know how to play a certain game, one of your friends can choose. Just search the internet and you will surely find a video or written instructions that will get you up to snuff.

Bocce: If you don't live near a bocce court, don't worry. You can purchase a set of lawn bocce balls, which you can either play in your own backyard or at any public park or friend's yard. You will find eight balls in a set (four of one color or pattern and four of another) and one small white ball called the *pallino*. The game can be played with either two or four players, and the object is to see which side gets their bocce balls closest to the *pallino*. The first team to reach twelve points wins.

Italian card games: A deck of Italian cards can be purchased either online or at most Italian food stores at the checkout aisle with other last-minute items. Instructions will come with the cards, although they are also freely available on the internet or via video on YouTube. The most popular Italian card games are *briscola*, *tressette*, and *scopa*. Learning new games also keeps our brains sharp!

Tombola: In Italy, the bingo-like game of tombola is typically played with family members of all generations at Christmastime, but it can really be played at any time of the year, especially when inclement weather drives people to stay indoors.

Sports night: Pick a sport you and your friends are already fans of or one that you would like to learn more about, and have every-body bring their favorite snacks to share and root for your teams together. It doesn't matter if it's a soccer match, Formula 1 race, tennis championship, or the Olympic Games. Being a spectator to an exciting sports game is invigorating and fun.

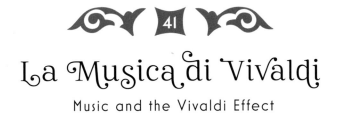

La Musica di Vivaldi

Music and the Vivaldi Effect

If I were to document only Italy's musical contributions to the world, I could fill multiple volumes. One Italian musical treasure was Antonio Vivaldi (1678–1741), or "*il prete rosso*" (the red priest) as he was called because of the color of his hair. Despite his extraordinary musical accomplishments, fame, and society's admiration, the priest turned composer was buried in a pauper's grave and his music quickly forgotten. It would be centuries before scholars rediscovered his scores and redeemed his works for all to enjoy. Now we can barely avoid hearing "La primavera" ("Spring" from *The Four Seasons*), even reduced in certain circumstances to background elevator music or what you might hear when put on hold as you wait for a live customer service representative on the phone.

Vivaldi was a Roman Catholic priest, a violin virtuoso, and a prolific composer who took bold creative risks, often creating a sharp division between those who were intrigued by his musical innovations, which often veered from the established rules of baroque, and those who disdained it. Father Vivaldi earned fame and admiration while teaching music and composition at a Venetian girls' orphanage. Ending in 1723, he wrote a series, *Il cimento dell'armonia e dell'invenzione* (The trial of harmony and invention), that included *The Four Seasons* (*Le quattro stagioni*). Each season ("Spring," "Summer," "Autumn," "Winter") was accompanied by an original sonnet, separated into thirds to go along with the three movements (fast-slow-fast) of the concerto format. The sonnets, to be read while listening to the music, beg us to hear the compelling sounds of each season, stunningly expressed by instruments of the string orchestra. We can actually experience the wonder of birds chirping, breezes blowing, dogs barking, and impending thunderstorms approaching.

Vivaldi's compositions are masterpieces to be enjoyed in their own right, but in recent years, researchers have chosen his compositions to examine the effect of music therapy on the cognitive performance of both healthy older adults as well as patients with Alzheimer's disease. The results have been consistently promising. Some call it "the Vivaldi effect." In one study, listening to an excerpt of *The Four Seasons* led to an improvement in attention and performance on category fluency tasks (i.e., naming as many examples as one can in a particular category within a minute) for both Alzheimer's and non-Alzheimer's participants.

Since memory impairment is one of the first signs of Alzheimer's disease, retaining autobiographical memory is crucial. Research findings in this area also showed Vivaldi excerpts helped participants with mild Alzheimer's to remember more about their own past—which is no small thing, since personal memories over the arc of our lives compose our self-concept and help us maintain a cohesive identity. In this study, participants with mild Alzheimer's were seen on two occasions. Both times, their recall was measured in an autobiographical memory interview. The background music on one visit was Vivaldi's "Spring" movement from *The Four Seasons*. On the other visit, there would be no music during the interview. Results showed a significant reduction in anxiety and a higher autobiographical memory recall in the music condition.

Despite physical or cognitive limitations, humans seem to have an innate ability to respond to music. Music can help us relax, feel happier and less anxious, and in general enhance our quality of life. One study examined cognitive performance in two working memory tasks in healthy older adults (ages seventy-three to eighty-six). The participants were presented tasks involving digit span (number sequence repetition) and phonemic fluency (a timed test naming as many words as possible starting with a specific letter), while in the background, there would be Vivaldi's music, white noise, or no music (repeated measures design). Performance was strongest when participants were completing tasks to the background music of Vivaldi's "Spring." It appears that this music enhanced mood and attention and also facilitated successful task completion.

Studies continue to be published exploring the efficacy of music and music therapy on behavioral and psychological symptoms of dementia. In fact, a thorough review by the Italian Psychogeriatric Association led to the recommendation that interventions with music can be considered a meaningful support in the management of these symptoms.

Is the therapeutic effect of music in older adults specific only to Vivaldi compositions? Probably not. Some studies have shown that one's preferred music might have the same effect, but certainly this eighteenth-century red-haired maestro left a powerful legacy—not only with respect to the world of music but to the world in general by virtue of the therapeutic effects of his masterpieces.

HOW TO MAKE YOUR OWN MUSIC

You don't have to be experiencing dementia to benefit from music. Even babies, before they learn to walk, will hang on to the side of their crib or play-pen and bob up and down to the beat of music. Educators find that certain music has a positive effect on student learning. When we grow older, certain songs provide a backdrop to the important events of our lives and a memory for the years ahead.

Have you always wanted to sing, play an instrument, or write a song? Did you once play an instrument but then had to let it go for one reason or another? Listening to music is therapeutic and uplifting, but making your own music can be even more satisfying. Today there are many internet courses in all aspects of music. Learn to sing, play an instrument, or dance. Do some research, read the reviews, and take action to make music a greater part of your life.

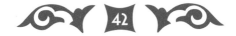

I Gatti dell'Antica Roma

The Lessons of Ancient Roman Cats

My grandmother Angelina had a best friend whom she called "Brrrownie" (pronounced with a trilled *r*). He was a brown-and-white-striped feline who understood only Italian. As a kid, whenever I visited *nonna*, Brownie would appear from wherever he was in the house at the first sound of my voice. I would tie up a bit of paper with string to make a lure and drag it around the kitchen table, Brownie chasing after it. When my grandmother had enough of the commotion, she would call Brownie in her native dialect, "*Vena ca*," and immediately the cat obeyed. It was time to get back to his official household duty of keeping the mice away from the wooden barrels in the wine cellar.

Italians have a long-standing relationship with cats, and if you go to Italy, you will notice thousands of both domesticated and feral cats, some cared for in designated cat colonies, such as the one in the little Sardinian coastal village of Su Pallosu, where volunteers care for and feed them and tourists come to admire them. Italy in general has almost eight million domesticated cats, according to Statista. In Rome alone there are about two thousand feral cat colonies, with approximately three hundred thousand cats living in them!

Cats have a mystical aura. They are mysterious, somewhat regal, and fiercely independent, which is why the ancient Romans had a fickle relationship with them. Dogs were originally the preferred companions, because of their loyalty, obedience, and ability to hunt. Eventually, however, the Egyptian almost cult-like worship of cats came to influence Roman attitudes, and cats came to be seen in a more positive light, valued for their usefulness in keeping mice and rats away from the soldiers' food and armor. With the spread of the Roman Empire, images of cats were seen on mosaics, banners of the Roman Legions, and tombstones. Cats not only accompanied the soldiers everywhere but also were found on Roman ships that sailed to meet Chinese merchants in Ceylon to trade.

Today you will see stray cats throughout the Roman ruins and the Roman Colosseum. Over three hundred thousand cats now live in Rome alone—half of which are domestic pets, the other half strays. You will see them stretching, sunning themselves, and hiding under shady alcoves on the streets and in cat colonies, which are protected by Roman law. A *gattara* is someone who looks after cats in their protected colonies. Local authorities take care of the free neutering of their feline populations, and harming cats is illegal in Italy.

While there is no doubt that Italy has a big heart when it comes to caring for cats, whether at home or on the streets, simply observing these curious animals can teach us a few important lessons on how to live la dolce vita.

FIVE SELF-CARE LESSONS FROM THE ROMAN CATS

We often think we are the ones to teach our animals important behaviors. If we stop and think a moment, however, we will discover the important life lessons that animals have a way of teaching us.

- ✿ Be inquisitive. Pursue your curiosity and make new discoveries in familiar settings.

- ✿ Nurture your body daily by stretching, stepping lightly, basking in a sunny window, and following a meticulous grooming routine.

- ✿ Eat just enough to feel satisfied and energized, not stuffed and tired.

- ✿ Maintain your sense of independence. You have all the answers you need inside you.

- ✿ Be of service to others, like the cats who kept rodents from eating the Roman soldiers' food and armor.

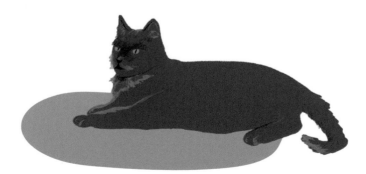

L'Automobile

The Italian Car and Insights for Success

Italians are unabashedly all about aesthetics. Made-in-Italy craftmanship is apparent in Italy's fashion, art, engineering, architecture, and of course in their cars, which are fast, gracefully designed, and a source of envy for anyone who has ever had a dream of owning a Lancia, Bugatti, Lamborghini, Maserati, Ferrari, Alfa Romeo, or even a FIAT.

The Italian driver is attentive to the sleek lines, the feel, the sound—and the speed—of a well-constructed Italian car, which inevitably becomes an extension of its owner. Not surprisingly, a good percentage of Italy's people will admit they are avid fans of motorsports. Italy has a rich history of auto racing, and they love their fast *automobili.*

The Alfa Romeo originally displayed a *quadrifoglio,* or four-leaf clover, as an emblem of good luck. The Alfa company, started in 1910, has achieved ten Grand Prix wins, has appeared in Super Bowl ads, and is also a popular Italian car choice outside Italy, as is FIAT (Fabbrica Italiana Automobili Torino), launched in 1900 when Giovanni Agnelli opened the first FIAT factory in Torino, Italy, and the first U.S. factory in 1908. FIAT was one of the most popular street cars in Italy for an entire century, and although not particularly a racing car, it has won European Car of the Year multiple times.

Maserati achieved nine Grand Prix wins and was originally a product of three sons of a railway worker who launched the company in Bologna in 1914;

another brother, who had no particular interest in automobiles but rather a passion for living an artist's life, became the designer of the Maserati logo—the trident (a three-pronged spear, in ancient Roman and Greek mythology signifying domination of the seas).

The Italian race car is much lighter, sleeker, more nimble at turning corners, and lower to the ground than most American racing cars. Yet the car itself is only half of a successful win; the driver is the other 50 percent of the equation. While not everyone is cut out to be a race car driver, we can glean a few important insights from a world-renowned Italian race car driver like Mario Andretti.

Researchers have found that race car drivers are thrill-seekers but not risk-takers. The experience of the thrill incites the brain to release feel-good chemicals, including endorphins, dopamine, and adrenaline. However, to take "risks" when driving up to two hundred miles an hour can result in disaster. Andretti, in an interview with Dr. Patrick Cohn, revealed that one must stay focused and have an intense ability to concentrate in addition to self-confidence and the belief that they are going to win and will accept no less. Andretti was born in Montona, Istria (which was then part of Italy), and became a motorsport legend, winning races in Formula 1, IndyCar, and NASCAR.

While most of us will not become race car drivers and will hopefully not consider speed limits, stop signs, and traffic lights to be mere suggestions, which Italians have been described as doing, there are a few valuable insights Andretti shared on the topic of success, not only in the motorsports world but in any field.

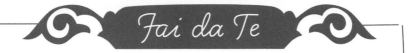

Fai da Te

SUCCESS TIPS FROM A WORLD-RENOWNED ITALIAN RACE CAR WINNER

Italians love car-racing competitions. Here are some winning tips that go beyond the sport and can be useful in helping you obtain what you desire in your life.

❀ Start with a desire.

❀ Let your desire fuel your passion.

❀ Work hard and be motivated to win.

❀ Have the mindset of confidence in approaching your task.

❀ Set very high goals, and believe you can reach them.

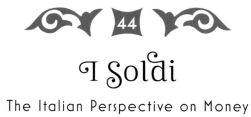

I Soldi

The Italian Perspective on Money

Classic fairy tales often mirror cultural perspectives and attitudes. In the famous Italian fairy tale *Pinocchio*, the marionette is given five gold coins to buy an ABC schoolbook, which his poor father had to sell his tattered coat for to afford. On the way to buy the book, however, Pinocchio meets a cunning fox and a cat who convinces him that if he buried his coins in a certain field, they will grow into a money tree, multiplying his wealth many times over without having to work for it. Unfortunately, the fox and cat steal his money, and Pinocchio quickly learns that the only way to rescue his father and himself from poverty is to do it the old-fashioned way: through hard physical work. This little story illustrates the Italian belief that earning money requires hard work. But on the other hand, Italians believe that the purpose of money is not to amass it to build wealth but rather to enjoy the fruits of one's labor. While they wisely put some of their earnings aside for a rainy day, the rest should be used to enjoy life and to be generous with family and friends with whatever they have.

A fascinating study published in *American Behavioral Scientist* compared Italians with the Swiss on the meaning of money. The authors studied fairy tales, folklore, literature, and interviews from the two cultures. Overall, they found the Swiss preferred not to talk about money or one's salary. In Italy, both Catholicism and communism influenced the thinking that excessive wealth had an evil connotation; however, money earned through hard work and shared with others was a redeeming factor, as was the belief that money is the means to an end and not the end itself.

The researchers found that while to the Swiss, investing and holding on to one's money to watch it grow was the priority, for Italians, it was more important to enjoy the money one had. When survey respondents were asked what they would do with their money if they were to suddenly become rich, Italians said they would splurge or buy something nice for family or friends. When asked the same question, the Swiss stated they would save or invest.

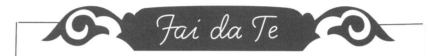

Fai da Te

AN ITALIAN BALANCED APPROACH TO MONEY

Italians work hard for what they earn, but as important as one's work is, it takes a back seat to celebratory living. Here are some ways you can adopt the same mindset.

- ❅ Work hard and always do your best if you have a job that provides for your needs.

- ❅ Plan out how much money you need to put aside for emergencies; then do so regularly.

- ❅ Be generous and thoughtful with your friends and family by giving them small gifts, taking them to dinner, or gifting them money when they need it.

- ❅ Splurge on yourself occasionally.

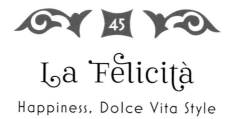

La Felicità

Happiness, Dolce Vita Style

In 1982, an Italian pop song called *"Felicità"* ("Happiness") was made famous by the then husband and wife team of Al Bano and Romina Power. The lyrics capture the essence of the Italian philosophy of living a dolce vita. Happiness is found in ordinary simple pleasures. Beyond having enough money to pay the bills, no amount of money or possessions brings more happiness than the joy of a balanced, uncomplicated life surrounded by the people who love and care about you.

The ancient Roman definition of happiness comes from the writings of the Stoic philosopher Seneca, whose treatise "The Happy Life" emphasizes peace of mind and lasting tranquility, which one gleans from the soul, not in the human flesh. Such a soul is truthful, honorable, and kind. If we want to live happy and tranquilly, we must display these characteristics in thought, word, and deed.

Felicità also means focusing on the good in life and not dwelling on what doesn't make us happy. In 2014, over ten million Italians sat riveted to their television sets as Academy Award–winning actor Roberto Benigni of *La vita è bella* (*Life Is Beautiful*) gave a one-man show with a contemporary interpretation of the Ten Commandments (*I dieci comandamenti*). Pope Francis called the actor to personally thank him for bringing the commandments back into the homes of millions. One of the topics of his impassioned and moving monologue focused on our lifelong search for happiness. "We are always looking for it," Benigni observed, and "we must never stop seeking it till the day we die." However, he claimed, it is also true that we were given the gift of happiness the moment we were born and may have just forgotten that we still have this gift. "We search high and low, we empty all our closets, our drawers, our shelves in search of happiness, but we need only look into our own souls—it is right there. It never left," said the actor. In other words, happiness comes from *within* us.

Benigni's perspective is not terribly different from that of one of Italy's most respected psychiatrists and authors, Dr. Raffaele Morelli. In his book *La felicità è qui* (*Happiness Is Here*), he uses the analogy of the flower when answering the question "What is happiness?" We should not delude ourselves into thinking people can be happy all the time. Although we may try to fight aging, for instance, we are a part of nature, like the flower that loses its petals in winter. It is not unhappy because it is losing its petals, but from "cosmic sadness" comes a joy in the ability to embrace the phases of the natural cycle.

Happiness is not about the external. It is not about how we look, what objects we have, how much money we make, or what people say about us. "A spider," said Dr. Morelli, "makes a beautiful spider web out of instinct." We too have the instinctual power to be happy. We rediscover it when we get back in touch with our passions or simply ask ourselves, "What gives me joy?" Happiness is not something you get by forcing it or by resisting reality. It is about accepting what is with tranquility, navigating life's ups and downs serenely, and being in harmony with all aspects of one's life.

And then, of course, there is pizza. According to a survey conducted by the Italian research firm Doxa, a majority of survey respondents, when asked what makes them happy, reported that a good pizza does the trick. Presumably, that would likewise extend to a bowl of pasta, an Italian gelato, or even "a good supply of books and corn planned for the year," as described in the epistolary of the Roman poet Horace on how to be content.

Living la dolce vita is focusing your mental and physical radar on the little joys that make life so extraordinary.

Fai da Te

HAPPINESS SUMMARY

A few lessons on happiness in the land of dolce vita are as follows:

❁ Believe in yourself as the creator of your own happiness. Know that it does not depend on what you have or don't have.

❁ Accept life with all its ups and downs. No one is happy every minute of every day.

❁ Reflect on whatever it is you are passionate about. Maybe it is a hobby you abandoned years ago, a subject you want to learn more about, or a business you always wanted to start. Pursue those passions, and happiness will follow.

❁ To live a tranquil life, be a pillar of truth, kindness, and authenticity. Know you have the power within you to experience peace and serenity no matter what others think or do.

❁ Be a role model for happiness. Just as a yawn is contagious, when you are in the company of someone who is happy, you feel happy too. That is a gift you can spread to others.

❁ Enjoy a good pizza.

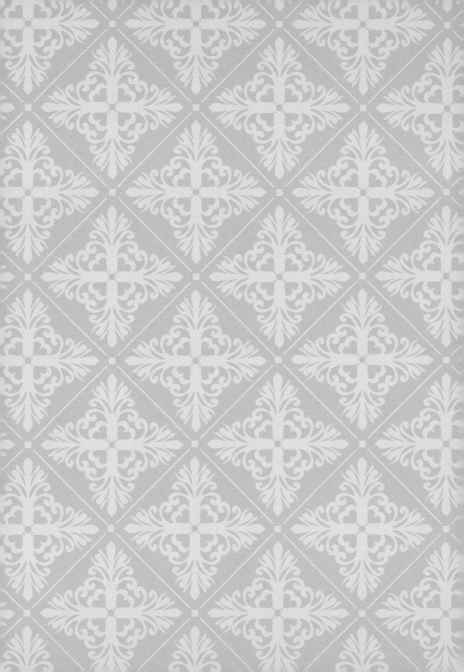

FAQ: The Italian *Dolce Vita* and How You Can Live the Sweet Life Too

Q: Didn't the original intent of the term *dolce vita*, conveyed in the famous film with Marcello Mastroianni and Anita Ekberg, refer to a period in Italy that was not so "dolce"?

A: In the film, as Rome was recovering from World War II, the country was in a phase of economic boom. The protagonist was in constant pursuit of pleasure, with an attitude of apathy and lack of meaning. Today, people associate the term *dolce vita* with a life of beauty, a life that Italians—despite the dark side of the human condition—have managed to attain through slow living, enjoyment of small pleasures, family, friends, food, wine, gelato, music, local fairs, simple picnics, and what are called the *piccole-grandi cose della vita* (the small yet great joys in life).

Q: I don't have much money for extras. No Ferrari for me, no Gucci handbag, no Ferragamo shoes. How am I supposed to get that feeling of the Italian dolce vita?

A: Most Italians don't have the luxuries you mention either. As in the story I told about my grandfather, the shoemaker, he was happy to earn enough to keep up with his bills, as he gave most of his inventory away. His wealth, he always said, was his three children, like three million dollars. It was his afternoon *caffè*, his *pane e cioccolato*, or the times his grandchildren read letters from the "old country" with him. You don't need luxury items to live the sweet life or to live like an Italian. I recently made a visit to an Italian novelty store and saw items priced at levels Italians in Italy would never purchase. The dolce vita is not about things. It is about experiences.

Q: **My life is too busy to live a dolce vita. I barely have time to breathe, let alone stop and notice a sunrise or a flower growing or enjoy a thunderstorm that lends itself to a rainbow.**

A: Slow living starts with a promise you make to yourself, a promise that you will be the guardian of your own well-being. Rushing through life will have you missing the beauty that is all around you. That means you don't eat supper while going through a drive-through. You stop multitasking and devote your full attention to everything you are doing. You pause every few minutes to notice your surroundings and take a few deep, slow breaths. You allow yourself to stroll rather than racewalk to get from one place to another. When you start living slower (that doesn't mean a boring or unrealistic snail's pace), you are giving yourself the gift of time, which will suddenly seem longer, more leisurely, and less stressful.

Q: **I hate to cook but I love Italian food. Can't I just order out from Italian restaurants instead of making it myself?**

A: There is nothing more healthful and satisfying than making food from your own kitchen, where you can control all the ingredients that go into it. Italians are passionate about the process, not just the end result. You will often hear my Italian family singing while cooking together, making it a joyful and special occasion. Learn to love cooking by starting out with something simple and delicious. If you like pasta, here is one of my favorite easy recipes, which I learned from a very special friend on the Amalfi Coast.

Pasta with Cherry Tomatoes

INGREDIENTS

1 pound spaghetti

A few drizzles extra virgin olive oil

3 cloves garlic, finely minced

½ small fresh chili pepper, seeded and minced

1 pint cherry or grape tomatoes, halved

Grated Parmigiano Reggiano (according to your taste)

4 basil leaves, finely torn

DIRECTIONS

Fill a large pot with water, and add a tablespoon or two of salt. Bring it to a boil. When the water is bubbling, add the pasta, and cook according to the package, timing it for the al dente amount of time.

While the pasta is cooking, add the olive oil to a skillet, and heat over medium heat until hot but not burning. Add the garlic and pepper, and stir until the garlic is golden but not brown (or it will be bitter). This takes only a minute or so, so don't leave the stove.

Add the cherry tomato halves, and lightly smash down with a wooden spoon to help squeeze the juice from the tomatoes. Add a ladle or two of the salted water that your pasta is cooking in.

Drain the pasta, and combine with the tomato mixture. Toss with a handful of grated Parmigiano Reggiano and the torn basil leaves. Serve with a tossed green salad on the side and a slice of crusty Italian bread.

Enjoy the process and the finished product by sharing this dish with someone. If you start simple and perform each step with curiosity and wonder, you will begin to fall in love with cooking and the satisfaction—and better health—it can bring you.

Q: I have been so busy with my career that I suddenly realize I really have no friends. Sure, I talk to coworkers when I go to work, but they aren't really relationships that extend beyond the eight-hour day. You say Italians point to friends when describing what the dolce vita is for them, but I don't live near a lively piazza or in a community that comes together to the sound of its *campanella*. I feel like I have no one to really talk to.

A   You are right to point out that, especially in the big cities, Italy is a mosaic of public squares where people gather each evening, take a *passeggiata*, greet their neighbors, start new conversations, and hang out with friends old and new. A lot of times, our lives get so busy that we lose touch with friends, or they move or turn away. Realize that great people don't just show up at your door and ask if they can be your friend. True friendship takes time, attention, and effort. Figure out where to find the kind of people you would like to be around. These days, through social media, it is easy to find old classmates or people you may have lost touch with. Invite them to meet you for a cup of coffee or even a virtual video chat. Another venue for establishing relationships is your place of worship or a community center. You may not have a *campanella* gonging in the background cueing to a community event, but you can certainly get involved in a church, synagogue, or mosque where you can begin to feel a sense of belonging.

Friendships begin over common interests. Attend a lecture on a topic you are interested in or a musical performance at your local university. Join a cultural club (Italian or other), and attend meetings. If you like to dance, there are plenty of dance groups, some that begin with a lesson. Sometimes you must get out of your comfort zone, but the more you do so, the easier it will become. Then gradually you can see which potential friends make a good fit with what you are looking for.

Q: How can Italians love family so much when every family I know has issues? They fight, stop speaking, even become estranged from one another. Do Italians have a secret for family cohesiveness that I don't know about?

A: For Italians, family comes first, but that doesn't mean they don't have their share of family disagreements and problems like everyone else. What trumps any argument, however, is love, pure and simple. Rarely do I hear about close family members permanently becoming estranged from each other or being mean to each other. That is not to say it doesn't happen, as Italians are human too, and I don't want to encourage a fantasy that doesn't exist. However, among a family that keeps love and loyalty as the glue that holds them together, disagreements don't have the power to trump blood. With family, you accept the good *and* the bad. You learn lessons from both. No family is perfect, so don't fret over situations you have no control over.

Q: Italy is so beautiful. Its beaches, its sunlit fields, its mountains, its lakes. Also, it has the most breathtaking architecture, art treasures, gondolas, and coastlines. I don't live in Italy and can't just fly out there on a whim. Is it really possible to feel the experience of Italy if I don't have the beautiful Italian scenery around me?

A: I was once given a needlepoint that read "Bloom where you are planted." That says it all. The idea of the dolce vita is maximum enjoyment of each day of your life. That doesn't mean life is perfect, but it means you accept and are satisfied with the life you were given. No matter where you live, look for the beauty, or create some of your own. There is beauty in an autumn tree, in a child laughing, in an art museum, in the morning fog. You create beauty when you organize and decorate your home or cultivate a flower garden or listen to a playlist of beautiful songs. Beauty uplifts our mood and has a healing effect on negative emotions and even our physical health. You don't have to forfeit beauty because you don't live in a certain locale.

Q: If the dolce vita is about love and romance, what do I do if I'm single and have no luck in finding someone?

A: You are right. The *bel paese* is a love peninsula for sure. You see public displays of affection in every corner and on every cobblestone road. But Italians are no different from you and me. And everything in its own time. There are times when they don't have partners and times when they do. They don't panic, because opportunities to love and be loved are all around you. Love your children, your parents, your siblings, your cousins, your friends, your pets. Become the lighthouse that emanates love to the world around you.

Acknowledgments

First and foremost, I would like to thank my Sourcebooks editor Erin McClary, whose valuable professional insights and keen attention to detail played a crucial role in shaping *45 Ways to Live Like an Italian*.

My deepest gratitude to the following top-notch team at Sourcebooks, whose important individual contributions have helped to make this book the very best it could be before sending it out into the world:

Mille grazie to Emily Proano, production editor, whose skill in pulling this project together is not to be understated; Jillian Rahn, art director, who led the design of the book's magical cover and internals; Stephanie Rocha, laying out the full cover; Brittney Mmutle, marketing manager, without whom this book could not reach the readers who might benefit; and also freelancers Kimberly Glyder for the cover and internal illustrations and Lindsey Cleworth for the internal design.

A heartfelt "thank you" to Sourcebooks publisher Dominique Raccah, who ultimately makes the decision about which books are valuable enough to see the light of day. She believed in my first book, *Living La Dolce Vita*, and I couldn't be more honored that she also believes in the potential of *45 Ways to Live Like an Italian* to enrich lives.

I hasten to acknowledge my three amazing adult children, who could not help but be raised with an awareness and appreciation for their Italian heritage: Casey Mautner Power, Thomas C. Mautner, and Dennis A. Mautner, Esq.

I wish to thank my childhood friend, and best-selling author, Stephen Spignesi, for always being available to share his important insights.

To Tiziano Dossena, author and editorial director of *L'Idea Magazine*, who so enthusiastically welcomed my articles for his online publication and allow me the time off that I needed to write this book.

To my beloved cousin Angelo Zeoli and all of my precious relatives of Castelpagano (BN), who inspire me and provide a constant reminder of the gift of my Italian roots.

To my dear friend Chris McNeil, whose profound philosophical insights kept me grounded in moments of uncertainty.

To my beloved best friend and prolific author Dr. Martin Kantor, whose wit and brilliance I will never forget as long as I live. May you rest in peace. I miss you dearly.

Finally, to "Lawrence," and he knows why.

Notes

Introduction. The Italian Celebration of La Dolce Vita

Author Luigi Barzini once described: Luigi Barzini, *The Italians: A Full-Length Portrait Featuring Their Manners and Morals* (New York: Touchstone, 1996), ix.

Marcello Mastroianni's character: *La Dolce Vita*, directed by Federico Fellini (Astor Pictures Corporation, 1960).

we can control our thoughts: Marcus Aurelius, *The Meditations of Marcus Aurelius*, trans. George Long (London: Watkins, 2006), 143.

Chapter 1. Mangia Bene: Eating Well the Italian Way

"be your source of wellness": Leonardo da Vinci, *Leonardo's Notebooks: Writing and Art of the Great Master*, ed. H. Anna Suh (New York: Black Dog & Leventhal, 2005), 392.

ages thirty to fifty-nine: Elisabetta Moro, "The Mediterranean Diet: From Ancel Keys to the Present," Mediterranean Diet, 2018, http://en.unescomeddiet.com/formazione/strumenti-formativi/item/8-la-dieta-mediterranea-da-ancel-keys-ai-giorni-nostri-ii.

high cholesterol, and other diseases: M. Dinu et al., "Mediterranean Diet and Multiple Health Outcomes: An Umbrella Review of Meta-Analyses of Observational Studies and Randomized Trials," *European Journal of Clinical Nutrition* 72, no. 1 (2018): 30–43, https://doi.org/10.1038/ejcn.2017.58.

who ate a typical Western diet: Patricia A. Ford et al., "Intake of Mediterranean Foods Associated with Positive Affect and Low Negative Affect," *Journal of Psychosomatic Research* 74, no. 2 (February 2013): 142–48, https://doi.org/10.1016/j.jpsychores.2012.11.002.

adhered to a Mediterranean diet: Antonio Ventriglio et al., "Mediterranean Diet and Its Benefits on Health and Mental Health: A Literature Review," *Clinical Practice and Epidemiology in Mental Health* 16, no. S1 (July 2020): 156–64, https://doi.org/10.2174/1745017902016010156.

overall better mental health: M. Corezzi et al., "Mediterranean Diet and Mental Health in University Students: An Italian Cross-Sectional Study," *European Journal of Public Health* 30, no. S5 (September 2020): ckaa166.201, https://doi.org/10.1093/eurpub/ckaa166.201.

adherence to the Mediterranean: Rosario Ferrer-Cascales et al., "Higher Adherence to the Mediterranean Diet Is Related to More Subjective Happiness in Adolescents: The Role of

Health-Related Quality of Life," *Nutrients* 11, no. 3 (March 2019): 698, https://doi.org/10.3390/nu11030698.

Food and Agriculture Organization: Elisabetta Moro, "The Mediterranean Diet from Ancel Keys to the UNESCO Cultural Heritage. A Pattern of Sustainable Development between Myth and Reality," *Procedia—Social and Behavioral Sciences* 223 (June 2016): 655–61, https://doi.org/10.1016/j.sbspro.2016.05.380.

Chapter 2. La Dieta Flexitariana: Variations on Mediterranean Eating

vegan lifestyle approximately doubled: T. Ozbun, "Vegetarians and Vegans in Italy 2014–2022," Statista, August 26, 2022, https://www.statista.com/statistics/609983/vegetarians-and-vegans-in-italy/.

improve overall health: Neal D. Barnard et al., "The Effects of a Low-Fat, Plant-Based Dietary Intervention on Body Weight, Metabolism, and Insulin Sensitivity," *American Journal of Medicine* 118, no. 9 (September 2005): 991–97, https://doi.org/10.1016/j.amjmed.2005.03.039.

improvement in focus: Jill Schildhouse, "How a Plant-Based Diet Can Affect Your Mood," *Vegetarian Times*, December 1, 2020, https://www.vegetariantimes.com/health-nutrition/mental-health/how-a-plant-based-diet-can-affect-your-mood/.

health and have more energy: John McDougall and Mary McDougall, *The Starch Solution: Eat the Foods You Love, Regain Your Health, and Lose the Weight for Good!* (New York: Rodale, 2012), Front matter comment by Dr. Neal Barnard..

gaining momentum everywhere: Ines Testoni et al., "Representations of Death Among Italian Vegetarians: An Ethnographic Research on Environment, Disgust and Transcendence," *Europe's Journal of Psychology* 13, no. 3 (August 2017): 378–95, https://doi.org/10.5964/ejop.v13i3.1301.

nutrients influence mental states: Ford et al., "Intake of Mediterranean Foods."

vegan nor entirely vegetarian: Laura Girolami. "Cresce il numero di flexitariani, consumatori 'flessibili' e consapevoli" [The number of flexitarians, "flexible" and aware consumers, is growing], *Il Giornale del Cibo*, June 20, 2018, https://www.ilgiornaledelcibo.it/FLEXITARIANI/.

Chapter 3. La Pasta Funzionale: Pasta with a Function

COVID-19 lockdown in: "Pasta: The Consumption's Increase [sic] During the Lockdown," BVA Doxa, October 21, 2020, https://www.bva-doxa.com/en/pasta-the-consumptions-increase-during-the-lockdown/.

true of carbohydrate intake: John M. de Castro, "Macronutrient Relationships with Meal Patterns and Mood in the Spontaneous Feeding Behavior of Humans," *Physiology & Behavior* 39, no. 5 (1987): 561–69, https://doi.org/10.1016/0031-9384(87)90154-5.

atherosclerotic cardiovascular disease: Mengna Huang et al., "Pasta Meal Intake in Relation to Risks of Type 2 Diabetes and Atherosclerotic Cardiovascular Disease in Postmenopausal Women: Findings from the Women's Health Initiative," *BMJ Nutrition, Prevention & Health* 4, no. 1 (April 2021): 195–205, https://doi.org/10.1136/bmjnph-2020-000198.

as well as glycemic load: Giuseppe Di Pede et al., "Glycemic Index Values of Pasta Products: An Overview," *Foods* 10, no. 11 (2021): 2541, https://doi.org/10.3390/foods10112541.

physical health and mental health: "Mind & Mood," Harvard Medical School, accessed November 7, 2022, https://www.health.harvard.edu/topics/mind-and-mood.

novel pasta products: Nadia Palmieri et al., "An Italian Explorative Study of Willingness to Pay for a New Functional Pasta Featuring *Opuntia ficus indica*," *Agriculture* 11, no. 8 (July 2021): 701, https://doi.org/10.3390/agriculture11080701.

Chapter 4. L'Alimentazione Sarda: Eat Like a Sardinian for a Long Life

age one hundred or older: Dan Buettner, *The Blue Zones: 9 Lessons for Living Longer from the People Who've Lived the Longest*, 2nd ed. (Washington: National Geographic, 2012).

this Sardinian phenomenon: Michel Poulain, Gianni Pes, and Luisa Salaris, "A Population Where Men Live as Long as Women: Villagrande Strisaili, Sardinia," *Journal of Aging Research* 2011, (2011): 153756, https://doi.org/10.4061/2011/153756.

positive social relationships: Maria Chiara Fastame, Marilena Ruiu, and Ilaria Mulas, "Hedonic and Eudaimonic Well-Being in Late Adulthood: Lessons from Sardinia's Blue Zone," *Journal of Happiness Studies* 23, (2022): 713–26, https://doi.org/10.1007/s10902-021-00420-2.

greater levels of happiness: Neal Lathia et al., "Happier People Live More Active Lives: Using Smartphones to Link Happiness and Physical Activity," *PLoS ONE* 12, no. 1 (January 2017): e0160589, https://doi.org/10.1371/journal.pone.0160589.

Chapter 5. Pane e Cioccolato: A Snack of Bread and Chocolate = Nostalgia

connected to that experience: John S. Allen, "Food and Memory," *Harvard University Press* (blog), May 18, 2012, https://harvardpress.typepad.com/hup_publicity/2012/05/food-and-memory -john-allen.html.

"Indians of that country": Girolamo Benzoni, *History of the New World*, trans. and ed. W. H. Smyth (London: Hakluyt Society, 1857), 150.

chocolate to China: "The Italian Market Potential for Cocoa," CBI Ministry for Foreign Affairs, September 3, 2020, https://www.cbi.eu/market-information/cocoa-cocoa-products/italy /market-potential.

and improve brain function: Jamie Eske, "What Are the Benefits of Dark Chocolate?", Medical News Today, April 13, 2022, https://www.medicalnewstoday.com/articles/dark-chocolate.

improved in young adults: María Angeles Martín, Luis Goya, and Sonia de Pascual-Teresa, "Effect of Cocoa and Cocoa Products on Cognitive Performance in Young Adults," *Nutrients* 12, no. 12 (November 2020): 3691, https://doi.org/10.3390/nu12123691.

treatment of mild cognitive impairment: Rocco Salvatore Calabrò et al., "The Efficacy of Cocoa Polyphenols in the Treatment of Mild Cognitive Impairment: A Retrospective Study," *Medicina* 55, no. 5 (May 2019): 156, https://doi.org/10.3390/medicina55050156.

reduction in negative affect: Ji-Hee Shin et al., "Consumption of 85% Cocoa Dark Chocolate Improves Mood in Association with Gut Microbial Changes in Healthy Adults: A Randomized Controlled Trial," *Journal of Nutritional Biochemistry* 99, (January 2022): 108854, https://doi .org/10.1016/j.jnutbio.2021.108854.

Chapter 6. Le Bevande Italiane: What Italians Drink

effective in preventing both: "Compound Found in Red Wine Opens Door for New Treatments for Depression, Anxiety: Resveratrol, Found in Grape Skin, Shuts Down Depression-Causing Enzyme in Brain," ScienceDaily, July 19, 2019, https://www.sciencedaily.com /releases/2019/07/190729094553.htm.

than people who did not: Alan Leviton, "Coffee Consumers Are Less Likely than Others to Be Depressed: A Review of the Current Research on Coffee, Depression, and Depressive Symptoms," National Coffee Association, accessed November 7, 2022, https://www.ncausa.org /Portals/56/PDFs/Communication/20200504_Leviton_white_paper_final.pdf.

United States coming in fifth: Kate MacDonnell, "Coffee Consumption by Country," Coffee Affection, September 23, 2022, https://coffeeaffection.com/coffee-consumption-by-country/.

Chapter 7. La Merenda Italiana: Italian Snack Ideas

"with a constant diet of sweets": Pellegrino Artusi, *Science in the Kitchen and the Art of Eating Well* (Lorenzo da Ponte Italian Library) 2003. Toronto: University of Toronto Press (3rd ed.), 577.

four hundred young adults: Tamlin S. Conner et al., "On Carrots and Curiosity: Eating Fruit and Vegetables Is Associated with Greater Flourishing in Daily Life," *British Journal of Health Psychology* 20, no. 2 (May 2015): 413–27, https://doi.org/10.1111/bjhp.12113.

as chips and sweets: Conner et al., "On Carrots and Curiosity."

life satisfaction, and happiness: Deborah R. Wahl et al., "Healthy Food Choices Are Happy Food Choices: Evidence from a Real Life Sample Using Smartphone Based Assessments," *Scientific Reports* 7, no. 1 (December 2017): 17069, https://doi.org/10.1038/s41598-017-17262-9.

"injurious to the health": da Vinci, *Leonardo's Notebooks*, 302.

increase the feeling of happiness: Sharon Liao, "25 Easy Ways to Feel Great," *Arthritis Today* 28, no. 1 (2014): 34.

Chapter 8. Cibo di Strada: Italian Street Food

new era of Italian street food: Fabio Parasecoli, "Eating on the Go in Italy: Between *Cibo di Strada* and Street Food," *Food, Culture & Society* 24, no. 1 (January 2021): 112–26, https://doi.org/10.1080 /15528014.2020.1859901.

Gusti d'Italia lists some: "A Guide to Traditional Italian Street Food," *Gusti d'Italia* (blog), May 20, 2023. https://gustiditalia.com/en/a-guide-to-traditional-italian-street-food/.

Chapter 9. Il Ritmo Quotidiano: The Daily Rhythm

"hangs on tomorrow and loses today": Lucius Annaeus Seneca, *On the Shortness of Life*, trans. C. D. N. Costa (New York: Penguin, 1997), 13.

Chapter 10. Il Dolce Far Niente: The Sweetness of Doing Nothing

"good ordering of the mind": Aurelius, *Meditations*, 46.

lead to personal transformation: Abraham H. Maslow, *Toward a Psychology of Being* (Sublime Books, 2014), 67.

Chapter 11. La Pausa: The Importance of Taking a Break

psychological as well as physical benefits: "The Benefits of Napping," Washington Center for Women & Children's Wellness, accessed November 8, 2022, https://www.wcwcw.org/blog/the -benefits-of-napping.

"if I may have Italy": Michael A. Musmanno, *The Story of the Italians in American* (New York: Doubleday 1965), 255.

engaged in that platform: Morten Tromholt, "The Facebook Experiment: Quitting Facebook Leads to Higher Levels of Well-Being," *Cyberpsychology, Behavior, and Social Networking* 9, no. 11 (November 2016): 661–66, https://doi.org/10.1089/cyber.2016.0259.

Chapter 12. Attività per Felicità: Activity for Happiness

reduce stress, anxiety, and depression: Mohammed Abou Elmagd, "Benefits, Need and Importance of Daily Exercise," *International Journal of Physical Education, Sports and Health* 3, no. 5 (2016): 22–27, https://www.kheljournal.com/archives/?year=2016&vol=3&issue=5&part=A&ArticleId=577.

come back to exercising the mind: Lucius Annaeus Seneca, *Letters from a Stoic* (Cambridge: Vigeo Press, 2016), 24.

pavement-pounding routines: Sophia Loren, *Women & Beauty* (London: William Morrow, 1984), 122.

authority on this dance form: Alessandra Belloni (website), accessed November 8, 2022, https:// alessandrabelloni.com.

Chapter 13. Il Giardino: The Italian Garden

bel paese, especially among families: "Gardening in Italy—Statistics and Facts," Statista, September 12, 2022, https://www.statista.com/topics/6960/gardening-in-italy/#topicHeader_wrapper.

inevitable losses we experience: Theresa L. Scott, Barbara M. Masser, and Nancy A. Pachana, "Exploring the Health and Wellbeing Benefits of Gardening for Older Adults," *Ageing & Society* 35, no. 10 (2015): 2176–200, https://doi.org/10.1017/S0144686X14000865.

producers in the European Union: International Trade Association, "Italy-Country Commercial Guide" (2021), https://www.trade.gov/country-commercial-guides/italy-agricultural-sector.

plant, water, reap, and admire: Jane Clatworthy, Joe Hinds, and Paul Camic, "Gardening as a Mental Health Intervention: A Review," *Mental Health Review Journal* 18, no. 4 (2013): 214–25, https://doi .org/10.1108/MHRJ-02-2013-0007.

Chapter 14. La Tecnica del Pomodoro: How to Make Time for What You Need to Do

Pomodoro Technique was born: "The Pomodoro Technique," Francesco Cirillo (website), accessed November 8, 2022, https://francescocirillo.com/products/the-pomodoro-technique.

and after time management training: Alexander Häfner, Armin Stock, and Verena Oberst, "Decreasing Students' Stress through Time Management Training: An Intervention Study," *European Journal of Psychology of Education* 30, (2015): 81–94, https://doi.org/10.1007/s10212-014 -0229-2.

Chapter 15. Il Sorriso Italiano: The Italian Smile

movement of the mouth only: Rebecca Joy Stanborough, "Smiling with Your Eyes: What Exactly Is a Duchenne Smile?", Healthline, June 29, 2019, https://www.healthline.com/health/duchenne -smile.

facial feedback hypothesis: Nicholas A. Coles, Jeff T. Larsen, and Heather C. Lench, "A Meta-Analysis of the Facial Feedback Literature: Effects of Facial Feedback on Emotional Experience Are Small and Variable," *Psychological Bulletin* 145, no. 6 (June 2019): 610–51, https://doi .org/10.1037/bul0000194.

"and give chances to grow": Anna Scelzo et al., "Mixed-Methods Quantitative-Qualitative Study of 29 Nonagenarians and Centenarians in Rural Southern Italy: Focus on Positive Psychological Traits," *International Psychogeriatrics* 30, no. 1 (January 2018): 31–38, https://doi.org/10.1017 /S1041610217002721.

of the manipulated variations: Emanuela Liaci et al., "Mona Lisa Is Always Happy—and Only Sometimes Sad," *Scientific Reports* 7, (2017): 43511, https://doi.org/10.1038/srep43511.

Chapter 16. La Sprezzatura: Making the Difficult Look Easy

making the difficult look easy: Baldassare Castiglione, *The Book of the Courtier*, trans. George Bull (New York: Penguin Classics, 1976), 37.

"colloquial American delivery": Carlo Bernardini, *Enrico Fermi: His Work and Legacy* (New York: Springer, 2004), 391.

greater overall life satisfaction: Yolande van Zyl and Manilall Dhurup, "Self-Efficacy and Its Relationship with Satisfaction with Life and Happiness among University Students," *Journal of Psychology in Africa* 28, no. 5 (October 2018): 389–93, https://doi.org/10.1080/14330237.2018.15 28760.

Chapter 17. Le Parole: The Power of Words to Cultivate Serenity

community, and social settings: Roberto Assagioli, *The Act of Will* (Baltimore: Penguin Books, 1974), 38.

Chapter 18. La Moda Italiana: Italian Fashion

dressed in more flattering clothing: Neil Howlett et al., "The Influence of Clothing on First Impressions: Rapid and Positive Responses to Minor Changes in Male Attire," *Journal of Fashion Marketing and Management* 17, no. 1 (February 2013): 38–48, https://doi .org/10.1108/13612021311305128.

Chapter 19. I Segreti di Bellezza: Beauty Secrets of the Stars

to change your life: Piero Ferrucci, *La bellezza e l'anima: Come l'esperienza del bello cambia la nostra vita* [Beauty and the soul: how the experience of beauty changes our life] (Milan: Mondadori, 2017).

everywhere if we look for it: Piero Ferrucci, *Beauty and the Soul* (New York: Penguin, 2009), 15.

and psychological health: Eugene W. Mathes and Arnold Kahn, "Physical Attractiveness, Happiness, Neuroticism, and Self-Esteem," *Journal of Psychology* 90, no. 1 (1975): 27–30, https://doi.org/10.10 80/00223980.1975.9923921.

"and never give up": Martin Gani, "Interview with Claudia Cardinale," *Italy Magazine*, April 10, 2012, https://www.italymagazine.com/featured-story/interview-claudia-cardinale.

to clean the pores: Gina Lollobrigida, interview by Lydia Lane, 1959, https://neglectedvenus .wordpress.com/tag/gina-lollobrigida/.

Christian Dior's Hypnotic Poison: Sandra Raičević Petrović, "New Face of Dior Hypnotic Poison— Monica Bellucci," Fragrantica, accessed November 8, 2022, https://www.fragrantica.com/news /New-Face-of-Dior-Hypnotic-Poison-Monica-Bellucci-512.html.

beauty comes from the inside: Diego Dalla Palma, *La bellezza interiore* [Inner beauty] (Toronto: Sperling & Kupfer, 2006), 51.

Chapter 20. La Donna Italiana: The Italian Woman

life that require effort: Markham Heid, "Hard Work Is the Key to True Happiness (aka, Your Parents Were Right)," Medium, November 29, 2019, https://elemental.medium.com/hard-work-is-the -key-to-true-happiness-aka-your-parents-were-right-cfeb20bbe02a.

Chapter 21. I Rimedi da Cucina Italiana: Italian Kitchen Remedies

improve both health and appearance: *I miracolosi remedi della nonna* [Grandmother's miraculous remedies] (n.p.: RIZA, 2017), https://shopping.riza.it/riza-colletcion-i-miracolosi-rimedi-della -nonna.html.

and boost hydration: Annie Doyle, "11 Reasons to Add Vitamin C Serum to Your Skincare Routine," Healthline, August 19, 2022, https://www.healthline.com/health/beauty-skin-care/vitamin-c -serum-benefits.

you can get to a dentist: Joe Leech, "11 Proven Health Benefits of Garlic," Healthline, May 2, 2022, https://www.healthline.com/nutrition/11-proven-health-benefits-of-garlic.

Chapter 22. I Gesti: The Art and Value of Italian Hand Gestures

"the inflection of the voice": Marcus Tullius Cicero, *De Oratore*, trans. Jakob Wisse (New York: Oxford University Press, 2001), 37.

the nose while speaking: Marcus Fabius Quintilianus, *Institutio Oratoria*, trans H. E. Butler (London: Forgotten Books, 2018), 309.

expert Dr. Isabella Poggi: Rachel Donaldo, "When Italians Chat, Hands and Fingers Do the Talking," *New York Times*, June 30, 2013, https://www.nytimes.com/2013/07/01/world/europe/when-italians-chat-hands-and-fingers-do-the-talking.html.

of Pompeii and Herculaneum: Andrea de Jorio, *Gesture in Naples and Gesture in Classical Antiquity: A Translation of Andrea de Jorio's* La mimica degli antichi investigata nel gestire napoletano, trans. Adam Kendon (Bloomington: Indiana University Press, 2000).

the children got a bit older: Jana M. Iverson et al., "Learning to Talk in a Gesture-Rich World: Early Communication in Italian vs. American Children," *First Language* 28, no. 2 (May 2008): 164–81, https://doi.org/10.1177/0142723707087736.

"imaginatively than any other people": Barzini, *Italians*, 62.

culture, or mother tongue: Luca Vullo, "The Italian Language of Gestures and the Power of Nonverbal Communication," Italian Innovators, September 20, 2021, YouTube video, 36:19, https://www.youtube.com/watch?v=1SbxrwbuH9Q.

predictors of a happy life: Thomas Oppong, "Good Social Relationships Are the Most Consistent Predictor of a Happy Life," Thrive Global, October 18, 2019, https://thriveglobal.com/stories/relationships-happiness-well-being-life-lessons/.

and communication disorders: Sharice Clough and Melissa C. Duff, "The Role of Gesture in Communication and Cognition: Implications for Understanding and Treating Neurogenic Communication Disorders," *Frontiers in Human Neuroscience*, August 11, 2020, https://doi.org/10.3389/fnhum.2020.00323.

Chapter 23. Consiglio sulla Vita Amoroso: Love Advice from the Bel Paese

to another human being: "Why Is Intimacy Important in Older Adults," National Council on Aging, December 15, 2021, https://www.ncoa.org/article/why-is-intimacy-important-in-older-adults.

increase in positive emotions: Adrienne Santos-Longhurst, "Why Is Oxytocin Known as the 'Love Hormone'? And 11 Other FAQs," Healthline, August 30, 2018, https://www.healthline.com/health/love-hormone.

"before, is tied tighter still": Veronica Franco, *Poems and Selected Letters*, ed. and trans. Ann Rosalind Jones and Margaret F. Rosenthal (Chicago: University of Chicago Press, 1999), 69.

"smoother than her own mirror": Ovid, *The Art of Love and Other Poems*, trans. J. H. Mozley (Cambridge: Harvard University Press, 1979), 7.

"be a fish in the stream": Ovid, *Art of Love*, 149.

"and good looks": ibid., 149.

"that you are feigning": ibid., 87.

mistaken for true love: Francesco Alberoni, *Il mistero dell'innamoramento* [The mystery of falling in love] (Milan: Rizzoli, 2003), 19.

definition in Buscaglia's view: Leo Buscaglia, *Amore* (Milano: Mondadori 1972), 107.

it comes to finding love: Silvano Arieti and James Arieti, *Love Can Be Found* (New York: Harcourt Brace Jovanovich, 1977), 107.

healing from a broken heart: Francesco Campione, *10 regole per guarire le ferite d'amore* [10 rules to heal the wounds of love] (Bologna: Taita, 2013), 21.

"think, to enjoy, to love": Brainy Quote, Marcus Aurelius, https://www.brainyquote.com/quotes/marcus_aurelius_132163.

Chapter 24. Fare Quattro Chiacchiere: The Italian Art of the Chitchat

humdrum day of routine: Daniel Goleman, *Emotional Intelligence: Why It Can Matter More Than IQ* (New York: Bantam, 1995), xix.

"the mind of the speaker": Aurelius, *Meditations*, 103.

powerful tools of communication: Dale Carnegie, *How to Win Friends and Influence People* (New York: Pocket Books 1998), 17.

"Really?" he replied: Jerome Hines, *Great Singers on Singing* (Brisbane: Limelight, 1987), 103.

Chapter 25. Le Parolacce: Italian Curse Words (If You Must)

about the content of their message: "Poise, Presence, and Passion," Corporate Communications Experts, accessed November 9, 2022, https://corporatecommunicationexperts.com.au/poise-presence-passion-3-tools-help-confident-effective/.

Chapter 26. Le Lezioni di Vita: Casanova's Lessons for a Passionate Life

"Creator's own divinity": Casanova, *History of My Life*, 26.

"meant to make us happy": ibid., 33.

"to love my teacher": ibid., 38.

Chapter 27. L'Amicizia: A Roman Perspective on Friendship

on this subject of all time: Marcus Tullius Cicero, *How to Be a Friend: An Ancient Guide to True Friendship*, trans. Philip Freeman (Princeton: Princeton University Press, 2018).

insights on the subject: Lucius Annaeus Seneca, *Letters from a Stoic*.

Chapter 28. Il Galateo: Italian Rules of Etiquette

Giovanni della Casa in 1558: Giovanni della Casa, *Galateo*, Italian edition (Rome: Flower-ed, 2018).

Chapter 29. La Saggezza Italiana: Italian Wisdom for Living

"be a wonderful part of life": Marcus Tullius Cicero, *How to Grow Old: Wisdom for the Second Half of Life*, trans. Philip Freeman (Princeton: Princeton University Press, 2016), xii.

"spellbound by her beauty": Ovid, *Art of Love*, 87.

Chapter 30. La Meditazione di Passaggio: The Power of Passage Meditation

inspirational reading passage: D. Oman, J. Hedberg, and C. E. Thoresen, "Passage Meditation Reduces Perceived Stress in Health Professionals: A Randomized, Controlled Trial," *Journal of Consulting and Clinical Psychology* 74, no. 4 (August 2006): 714–19, https://doi.org/10.1037/0022 -006X.74.4.714.

and error from direct experience: Albert Bandura, *Social Learning Theory* (Hoboken, NJ: Prentice Hall, 1976).

went in part like this: Valerio Albisetti, *Come attraversare la sofferenza e uscirne più forte* [How to overcome suffering and come out of it stronger] (Milan: Paoline Libri, 2016), 20.

Chapter 31. La Creatività: The Gift of Creative Genius

"yields to stern resolve": da Vinci, *Leonardo's Notebooks*, 302.

Chapter 32. I Santi: The Italian Veneration of Saints

chalice, heart, or ladder: Italian American Museum of Los Angeles, "St. Joseph's Tables Take Us Back to Where It All Began," Italian Sons and Daughters of America, March 10, 2020, https:// orderisda.org/culture/old-school/st-josephs-tables-represent-the-cultural-and-religious -traditions-of-our-culture/.

Encyclopedia of Saints: Tessa Paul, *The Complete Illustrated Encyclopedia of Saints: An Authoritative Guide to the Lives and Works of Over 500 Saints, with Expert Commentary and Over 500 Beautiful Paintings, Statues, and Icons* (Horsham, UK: Southwater Press, 2018).

Chapter 33. La Magia Italiana: Italian Magic

protection from harm: "Curses, Countercurses, Incantations, and More Penn Museum's New Exhibition: Exploring Magic in the Ancient World," *University of Pennsylvania Almanac* 62, no. 30 (April 12, 2016), https://almanac.upenn.edu/articles/curses-countercurses-incantations-and -more-penn-museums-new-exhibition-exploring-magic-in-the-an.

"less than faith": Charles Godfrey Leland, *Aradia or the Gospel of the Witches* (1899; repr. Whithorn, UK: Anodos Books, 2018), 2.

by the dominant culture: Sabina Magliocco, "Imagining the Strega: Folklore Reclamation and the Construction of Italian American Witchcraft," in *Performing Ecstasies: Music, Dance, and Ritual in the Mediterranean*, ed. Luisa Del Giudice and Nancy van Deusen, 277–301 (Ottawa: Institute of Mediaeval Music, 2005), https://www.academia.edu/171085/Imagining_the_Strega.

Chapter 34. Il Malocchio e Superstizioni Italiane: The Evil Eye and Other Italian Superstitions

labeled under the category: Michael E. Bell, "Mal occhio—Demonstration of How to Remove the Evil Eye (Italian Tradition)," Rhode Island Folklife Project collection, Library of Congress, November 29, 1979, https://www.loc.gov/item/afc1991022_mb_048/.

Eusapia Palladino (1854–1918): Francesco Paolo de Ceglio and Lorenzo Leporierie, "Becoming Eusapia, The Rise of the 'Diva of Scientists,'" *Science in Context* 33, no. 4 (2020): 441–71, https://doi.org/10.1017/S026988972100020X.

criminologist Cesare Lombroso: Simone Natale, "The Medium Goes to America: The Forgotten Story of Medium Eusapia Palladino and Her Séance Tour of the United States," *History Today* 66, no. 5 (May 2016), https://www.historytoday.com/history-matters/medium-goes-to-america.

and watching over them: Paige Whitley, "Psychic Mediums," *Psychology of Extraordinary Beliefs* (blog), March 8, 2018, https://u.osu.edu/vanzandt/2018/03/08/psychic-mediums-2/.

awareness and inner guide: Lisa Held, "Psychic Mediums Are the New Wellness Coaches," *New York Times*, March 19, 2019, https://www.nytimes.com/2019/03/19/style/wellness-mediums.html.

Chapter 35. L'Arte di Arrangiarsi: The Art of Getting By

possibly prevent depression: Christopher Bergland, "More Evidence That Physical Activity Keeps Depression at Bay," *Psychology Today*, January 24, 2019, https://www.psychologytoday.com/us/blog/the-athletes-way/201901/more-evidence-physical-activity-keeps-depression-bay.

Chapter 36. La Famiglia: Italy as a Mosaic of Families

"together instinctually like ants": Barzini, *Italians*, 190.

general better mental health: Patricia A. Thomas, Hui Liu, and Debra Umberson, "Family Relationships and Well-Being," *Innovation in Aging* 1, no. 3 (November 2017): igx025, https://doi.org/10.1093/geroni/igx025.

taught him about life: Aurelius, *Meditations*, 7.

Chapter 37. La Casa Italiana: The Italian Home

"our joy of living": Ferrucci, *Beauty and the Soul*, 176.

four hours for Americans: Deborah Ball, "Women in Italy Like to Clean but Shun the Quick and Easy," *Wall Street Journal*, April 25, 2006, https://www.wsj.com/articles/SB114593112611534922.

in many Italian households: Maddalena De Bernardi, "*Tutte le virtù da riscoprire del sapone di Marsiglia*" [All the virtues to be rediscovered of Marseille soap], *Donna Moderna*, September 10, 2021, https://www.donnamoderna.com/ambiente/11-modi-per-usare-sapone-marsiglia.

Chapter 38. Il Cane Italiano: The Italian Dog

health by encouraging exercise: A. R. McConnell et al., "Friends with Benefits: On the Positive Consequences of Pet Ownership," *Journal of Personality and Social Psychology* 101, no. 6 (2011): 1239–52, https://doi.org/10.1037/a0024506.

than in the United States: Sirkku Sarenbo and P. Andreas Svensson, "Bitten or Struck by Dog: A Rising Number of Fatalities in Europe, 1995–2016," *Forensic Science International* 318, (January 2021): 110592, https://doi.org/10.1016/j.forsciint.2020.110592.

of dogs for different purposes: Marco Zedda et al., "Ancient Pompeian Dogs? Morphological and Morphometric Evidence for Different Canine Populations," *Anatomia Histologia Embryologia* 35, no. 5 (October 2006): 319–324, https://doi.org/10.1111/j.1439-0264.2006.00687.x.

households include cats: "Share of Households Owning at Least One Cat or Dog in Italy from 2014 to 2021," Statista, 2022, https://www.statista.com/statistics/517022/households-owning-cats-dogs-europe-italy/.

members of the family: "Pet's Life," BVA Doxa, May 16, 2019, https://www.bva-doxa.com/en/pets-life/.

avoid frightening animals: "Rome Bans New Year's Eve Fireworks," *Wanted in Rome*, December 30, 2021, https://www.wantedinrome.com/news/rome-bans-new-years-eve-fireworks.html.

yoga class if they wish: "Bau Beach: Rome's Beach Designated Exclusively for Dogs," *Wanted in Rome*, April 26, 2018, https://www.wantedinrome.com/yellowpage/bau-beach-romes-beach-designated-exclusively-for-dogs.html.

food and a place to sleep: Guy Davies, "IKEA in Italy Welcomes Stray Dogs This Winter," ABC News, November 22, 2018, https://abcnews.go.com/International/ikea-italy-welcomes-stray-dogs-winter/story?id=59315315.

for another living being: Caren Osten, "How Dogs Drive Emotional Well-Being," *Psychology Today*, April 18, 2018, https://www.psychologytoday.com/us/blog/the-right-balance/201804/how-dogs-drive-emotional-well-being.

Chapter 39. I Piccoli Piaceri: The Small Pleasures

frankly, I could believe it: "Nespole Fruit Season," Rove.me, March 31, 2021, https://rove.me/to/florence/nespole-fruit-season.

"thing and now at that": da Vinci, *Leonardo's Notebooks*, 11.

Chapter 40. Giochiamo!: The Italian Love of Games

percent of the land in Italy: "The Pareto Principle," Investopedia, updated April 7, 2022, https://www.investopedia.com/terms/p/paretoprinciple.asp.

video games regularly: James Batchelor, "It Took a Pandemic to Improve Acceptance of Video Games in Italy," Games Industry, April 15, 2021, https://www.gamesindustry.biz/it-took-a-pandemic-to-improve-acceptance-of-video-games-in-italy.

Chapter 41. La Musica di Vivaldi: Music and the Vivaldi Effect

"the Vivaldi effect": Nicola Mammarella, Beth Fairfield, and Cesare Cornoldi, "Does Music Enhance Cognitive Performance in Healthy Older Adults? The Vivaldi Effect," *Aging Clinical and Experimental Research* 19, no. 5 (October 2007): 394–99, https://doi.org/10.1007/BF03324720.

music of Vivaldi's "Spring": Mammarella, Fairfield, and Cornoldi, "The Vivaldi Effect."

management of these symptoms: A. Raglio et al., "Music, Music Therapy and Dementia: A Review of Literature and the Recommendations of the Italian Psychogeriatric Association," *Maturitas* 72, no. 4 (August 2012): 305–10, https://doi.org/10.1016/j.maturitas.2012.05.016.

Chapter 42. I Gatti dell'Antica Roma: The Lessons of Ancient Roman Cats

come to admire them: "A Colony of Cats on the Beach in Sardinia, Italy," Land of Cats, accessed November 10, 2022, https://www.landofcats.net/colony-cats-beach-sardinia-italy-2/.

cats, according to Statista: "Number of Cats in Italy from 2014–2021," Statista, June 2022, https://www.statista.com/statistics/516000/cat-population-europe-italy/.

300,000 cats living in them: "Cats in Rome, Italy!", Petrelocation, https://www.petrelocation.com/blog/post/cats-in-rome-italy.

protected by Roman law: "See Wild Cats Roam among the Ruins at a Cat Sanctuary in Rome," Travel Bliss Now, February 10, 2019, https://www.travelblissnow.com/cat-sanctuary-in-rome/.

Chapter 43. L'Automobile: The Italian Car and Insights for Success

first U.S. factory in 1908: "A Brief History of FIAT and Its Century of Automaking," FIAT of Scottsdale, April 24, 2015, https://www.fiatusaofscottsdale.com/blog/2015/april/24/a-brief-history-of-fiat.htm.

dopamine, and adrenaline: Jack Schafer, "Do You Have the Personality to Drive an Indy Car?", *Psychology Today*, May 21, 2015, https://www.psychologytoday.com/us/blog/let-their-words-do-the-talking/201505/do-you-have-the-personality-drive-indy-car.

and will accept no less: Patrick Cohn, "Interview with Mario Andretti on the Psychology of Racing," Peak Performance Sports, December 1, 2011, YouTube video, 15:24, https://www.youtube.com/watch?v=qfjFQ_g3W4s.

Chapter 44. I Soldi: The Italian Perspective on Money

tattered coat for to afford: Carlo Collodi, *Pinocchio: The Story of a Puppet* (Philadelphia: J. B. Lippincott Company, 1914).

on the meaning of money: Giovanna Dell'Orto and Kenneth O. Doyle, "Poveri Ma Belli: Meanings of Money in Italy and in Switzerland," *American Behavioral Scientist* 45, no. 2 (October 2001): 257–71, https://doi.org/10.1177/000276 40121957169.

Chapter 45. La Felicità: Happiness, Dolce Vita Style

not in the human flesh: Lucius Annaeus Seneca, in *Letters from a Stoic*. "On the Happy Life." Cambridge: Vigeo Press (2016): 202.

Ten Commandments (I dieci comandamenti): Silvia Fumarola. "Maratona Benigni, I Dieci comandamenti tutti in una sera." *La Repubblica*, May 8, 2020. https://www.repubblica.it/ spettacoli/tv-radio/2020/05/08/news/maratona_benigni_i_dieci_comandamenti_tutti_in _una_serata-255932971/.

phases of the natural cycle: Raffaele Morelli, *La felicità è qui* [Happiness is here] (Milan: Mondadori, 2012): 25.

good pizza does the trick: "Pizza Makes Italians Happy, Survey Finds," *Italy Magazine*, accessed November 10, 2022, https://www.italymagazine.com/dual-language/pizza-makes-italians -happy-survey-finds.

Horace on how to be content: Horace, *How to Be Content: An Ancient Poet's Guide for An Age of Excess*, trans. Stephen Harrison (Princeton: Princeton University Press, 2020), 51.

Index

M

N

About the Author

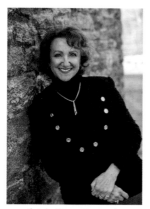

Photo by Kiernan Photography

Raeleen D'Agostino Mautner, PhD, is the author of *Living La Dolce Vita: Italian Secrets for Living a Happy, Passionate, and Well-Balanced Life* (Sourcebooks) and *Lemons into Limoncello: From Loss to Personal Renaissance with the Zest of Italy* (HCI Books). Both books were chosen as monthly selections by the Order of the Sons and Daughters of Italy in America. She has been recognized for her decades of work and contributions to the Italian American community, which include writing for such prestigious publications as *America Oggi*, the *Italian Tribune*, *Italian America*, *Psychology Today*, *Quirk's Marketing Research*, and the *Chicago Tribune*. She also writes a column for the foremost online publication for Italians throughout the world, *L'Idea Magazine*. Dr. Mautner has hosted and produced a popular radio show, *The Italian Art of Living Well*, at WNHU, has given many presentations (in Italy and throughout the United States), and has been interviewed on radio, TV, and print media on various topics that promote and maintain the positive tenets of Italian cultural traditions. Dr. Mautner has also been instrumental in helping combat negative stereotypes of Italians and Italian Americans.

She served as research director for the American Italian Defense Association and consulted for the memorandum of understanding between the Italian Consulate of NYC, Italian American Committee on Education, and the Connecticut Department of Education in creating the first Italian language resource center for Italian language teachers in the state of Connecticut. Dr. Mautner organized the first display of Italian American military heroes at the Newington campus of the Connecticut Veterans Healthcare Administration. She is the front singer for the Italian American band ENTERPRISE, which preserves and promotes the beautiful Italian and Italian American dance music of our heritage.

Sign up for her free newsletter at www.raeleenmautner.com, and join her Facebook author page (Raeleen Mautner, PhD Author) for the latest news on upcoming signings and events, including Facebook live talks.